**More praise for . . .**

*A Clinician's Guide to Controversial Illnesses*

"The book intelligently discusses both the medical and psychological aspects of this group of controversial and frustrating illnesses. It thoroughly reviews a wide spectrum of treatments, from mainstream to alternative. The sections on cognitive-behavioral therapy are practical, specific, and state-of-the-art. I highly recommend this book to practitioners who are trying to understand this group of illnesses, in order to help their affected patients."

  **–David C. Klonoff, MD, FACP,** Clinical Professor of Medicine,
  University of California at San Francisco

"Chronic fatigue syndrome (CFS), fibromyalgia (FMS), and multiple chemical sensitivities (MCS) once thought to be merely forms of malingering or minor psychological disturbances are now recognized as severe disorders with biological, psychological, and social components that profoundly incapacitate millions of Americans. Taylor, Friedberg, and Jason have crafted a scientifically-based but thoroughly readable book that brings together all that is known about the etiology, assessment, and multifaceted treatment of these disorders. Through standard forms, case studies, and a host of other materials, practitioners will learn exactly how to assess these disorders and apply treatment components that fully embrace the biopsychosocial model and psychoneuroimmunology. Empirically-validated and alternative biological and psychological treatments are carefully described and assessed for utility. As a practitioner – or if you are a person or have a friend or relative with one of these disorders – this book is absolutely essential reading."

  **–Richard A. Winett, PhD,** Heilig-Meyers Professor of Psychology,
  Director - Center for Research in Health Behavior, and Director of
  Clinical Training, Virginia Polytechnical Institute and State University

"This volume provides a clear, concise, and balanced overview of what we know and don't know about chronic fatigue syndrome and related disorders. *[The authors]* do an excellent job of melding empirical research and clinical wisdom. The case studies presented throughout the book nicely illustrate the authors' numerous valuable clinical insights. Taylor, Friedberg, and Jason's biopsychosocial approach holistically integrates material from diverse perspectives and points the way toward the types of comprehensive assessment, treatment, and education programs that are needed."

  **–David Glenwick, PhD,** Professor of Psychology, Fordham University

# A Clinician's Guide to Controversial Illnesses: Chronic Fatigue Syndrome, Fibromyalgia, and Multiple Chemical Sensitivities

RENÉE R. TAYLOR,
FRED FRIEDBERG, AND
LEONARD A. JASON

PROFESSIONAL RESOURCE PRESS
SARASOTA, FLORIDA

Published by
Professional Resource Press
(An imprint of the Professional Resource Exchange, Inc.)
Post Office Box 15560
Sarasota, FL 34277-1560

Printed in the United States of America

The copy editor for this book was David Anson, the managing editor was Debbie Fink, the production coordinator was Laurie Girsch, and Jami Stinnet created the cover.

**Library of Congress Cataloging-in-Publication Data**

Taylor, Renée R., date.
    A clinician's guide to controversial illnesses: chronic fatigue syndrome, fibromyalgia, and multiple chemical sensitivities / Renée R. Taylor, Fred Friedberg, and Leonard A. Jason.
        p. cm.
    Includes bibliographical references and index.
    ISBN 1-56887-068-X (alk. paper)
        1. Chronic fatigue syndrome. 2. Fibromyalgia. 3. Multiple chemical sensitivity. I. Friedberg, Fred. II. Jason, Leonard. III. Title.
        [DNLM: 1. Fatigue Syndrome, Chronic. 2. Fibromyalgia. 3. Multiple Chemical Sensitivity. WB 146 T245c 2001]
    RB150.F37 T39 2001
    616.0478--dc21

                                                            00-047837

# Dedication

May this book lead to the strengthening, nurturing, and validation of all individuals facing chronic fatigue syndrome, fibromyalgia, and multiple chemical sensitivities.

# Acknowledgments

We would like to thank a number of friends and colleagues whose insight, support, shared experiences, and constructive feedback made this book possible.

For sharing their wisdom regarding the multifaceted needs of individuals with these conditions, we wish to thank the following directors of local self-help organizations: Carole Howard of the Chicago CFS Association, Ron Gilbert of the Chronic Fatigue Syndrome Society of Illinois, and Sabrina Johnson of the Fibromyalgia Association Created for Education and Self-Help.

We would also like to thank a number of people who shared invaluable professional or personal experiences and insights regarding these conditions, including Morris Papernik, David Lipkin, Joyce Goodlatte, Judith Richman, Patricia Fennell, Doreen Salina, Audrius Plioplys, Sigita Plioplys, Harriet Melrose, Tony Albert, Joan Blake, Ken Lipman, Marty Greenberg, Dvorah Budnick, Randy Ravitts-Woodworth, Dawn Velligan, Patrick Holiday, Fabricio Balcazar, Chris Keys, and Stevan Hobfoll.

For their time, effort, and dedication to conducting research and promoting knowledge about these conditions, we wish to thank several individuals with whom we have worked closely at DePaul University, including Cara Kennedy and Heather Eisele who assisted us with editing needs, Constance Van der Eb, Susan Torres, Caroline King, Lynne Wagner, Karen Jordan, Mike Schoney, Nancy Carlin, Carrie Curie, Sharon Song, Radhika Chimata, Danielle Johnson, Adam Carrico, Trina Haney-Davis, and Jennifer Shlaes.

We would also like to extend a special thanks to Marjorie Piechowski, Denise Mattson, and Roxanne Brown Jahi of DePaul University for their ongoing support, dissemination, and promotion of our research and program development efforts.

Most importantly, we wish to thank the staff at Professional Resource Press, particularly Lawrence Ritt, Debra Fink, and Laurie Girsch for believing in this work and creating a much needed avenue for dissemination of information related to these conditions.

# Preface

A number of circumstances led to our decision to write this book, the most significant being the clear need for a practical and readable treatment guide for clinicians who are now encountering these patients in their practices. This book is an important resource for mental health professionals to better understand the complexities of diagnosing these conditions, identifying related psychological issues, and constructing effective treatment plans. This book also describes current theories of illness causation and perpetuation and promotes a broader understanding of a variety of approaches to treatment. Our hope is that it will serve as a timely and practical tool in helping clinicians navigate the unpredictable terrain that these conditions present.

*Renée R. Taylor*
*Fred Friedberg*
*Leonard A. Jason*

# Table of Contents

# A Clinician's Guide to Controversial Illnesses: Chronic Fatigue Syndrome, Fibromyalgia, and Multiple Chemical Sensitivities

# CHAPTER 1

# Introduction

Chronic fatigue syndrome (CFS), fibromyalgia (FMS), and multiple chemical sensitivities (MCS) are disabling conditions characterized by controversy over cause, nature, and treatment. In the absence of definitive diagnostic markers or laboratory tests to pinpoint an exact biomedical etiology, researchers and clinicians continue to struggle with some of the more puzzling and contradictory aspects of these conditions. This book is intended to provide health care professionals with both a clearer understanding of the complexities surrounding these conditions and a balanced perspective regarding integrative approaches to treatment.

Professionals working on behalf of individuals with CFS, FMS, and MCS should be aware of a number of shared challenges facing individuals with these conditions:

- *High variability of symptoms and impairments.* These illnesses exhibit enormous fluctuations in symptom severity and level of impairment between and within individuals. At one end of the spectrum of illness severity are relatively high-functioning individuals who are able to maintain full-time employment (although most likely at the expense of regular family, household, and social commitments). At the other end are patients who are homebound and must remain in bed for several hours during the day. Within individuals, there is considerable variability as well. For instance, a person who is homebound may feel well enough to leave the house, take short walks, and converse with others. On the other hand, a usually high-functioning individual may occasionally experience a "crash" and be unable to perform normal responsibilities for weeks or even months. Furthermore, sustained illness improvements or remissions that may last for months or years may end with prolonged periods of relapse. This heterogeneity is as baffling to patients as it is to the professionals involved in their treatment.

- *Curative treatments unavailable.* Many treatments attempted by individuals with controversial illnesses either do not work or are palliative only for selected symptoms. No curative medical interventions are available for any of these conditions. In part, this problem explains why many individuals with these conditions report negative experiences with treatment providers, and with physicians in particular. Many physicians rely solely on palliative pharmacologic agents, refer these patients for psychotherapy, or recommend no treatment whatsoever. Pharmacological management has been found to be helpful for certain individuals, particularly for those with FMS, while cognitive behavior therapy has been used effectively to help patients cope with their conditions. Multidisciplinary approaches that include medical supervision, nutritional counseling, physical therapy, social support, psychotherapy, and medication management may produce the most favorable outcomes. In addition to these approaches, many patients dissatisfied with Western medicine have utilized alternative treatments (covered in Chapter 5).

- *Increased prevalence in women.* Women comprise about 70% of patients with CFS, 90% of patients with FMS, and 75% of patients with MCS (Bell, Baldwin, & Schwartz, 1998; Jason, Richman, et al., 1999; Wolfe et al., 1995). Various cultural, psychological, and biological explanations have been offered for the gender imbalance in the affliction rate although no specific explanation has gained general acceptance. Some have argued that this "feminization" of these conditions has helped to undermine their social and political value.

- *High illness co-occurrence.* The level of co-occurrence of these illnesses within affected individuals appears to be high. Because these conditions show moderate symptomatic overlap with each other, some have suggested that they are variations of the same underlying disorder. However, factor analytic studies indicate that, despite commonalities in symptomatology, these illnesses can be considered distinct entities. From a clinical perspective, fatigue, pain, and chemical reactivity symptoms may each respond most favorably to somewhat different cognitive-behavioral and pharmacological interventions although the reactive emotional stress associated with all of these disorders can be treated with similar psychotherapeutic techniques. Leading researchers suggest that individuals with more than one of these conditions are significantly more impaired than those with one condition. Illness co-occurrence increases both the level of disability and the level of social stigma experienced by these individuals.

- *Low recovery rates.* These conditions are chronic for most individuals. In long-term prospective studies, only a minority (< 10%) of patients appear to achieve substantial recovery although a significant proportion will report some level of improvement over time (Joyce, Hotopf, & Wessely, 1997).
- *Multiple losses.* In severe cases, these disabilities can drain people of almost all economic and social resources and can leave a significant proportion unemployed or further disabled by an inappropriate employment situation. Those with fewest resources face severe economic hardship, social isolation, and lack of affordable housing. Those who are unable to work have had tremendous difficulty obtaining social security and disability benefits to help subsidize their income in spite of the fact that the social security administration recognizes CFS as a disability.
- *High psychiatric rates.* All of these chronic conditions are generally associated with higher than expected rates of psychiatric comorbidity as compared to the general population. However, some research suggests that rates of psychiatric disorder observed in individuals with these conditions are no higher than those observed in other medically ill populations. Moreover, the failure to identify symptomatic overlap between these illnesses and psychiatric disorders may result in misleading overestimations of psychiatric comorbidity in psychodiagnostic studies. It is likely that the psychiatric disorders that are observed in some individuals with these illnesses are triggered by the personal devastation resulting from symptoms, functional impairments, and resource losses. In a large-scale prevalence study of CFS, Jason, Richman, and associates (1999) found that a larger proportion of individuals with CFS

received a psychiatric diagnosis following fatigue onset as compared with before.

These commonalities among CFS, FMS, and MCS provide the rationale for grouping them together in this book. What applies to one will often apply to the others. We will use CFS as the model for understanding these controversial illnesses, but, when discussing FMS and MCS, we will highlight their unique features. Overall, this book provides the clinical practitioner with the information necessary to successfully engage, treat, and improve the quality of life for individuals with these conditions. Given the absence of effective medical treatments, the mental health professional can indeed offer hope and help to these patients.

## Case Definitions, Associated Symptoms, and Prevalence

Current prevalence data reveal that chronic fatigue syndrome (CFS) is one of the most prevalent and debilitating of all chronic health conditions, occurring in approximately .42% of the population, or 422 per 100,000 individuals, and affecting all aspects of life and functioning, including employment and activities of daily living (Jason, Richman, et al., 1999). This translates to approximately 800,000 U.S. citizens with this syndrome. Anderson and Ferrans (1997) conducted an investigation into the quality of life of persons with CFS. An analysis of the responses of 110 participants with CFS revealed that individuals with CFS reported significantly lower quality of life with respect to health and functioning, social, and economic aspects of life, as compared with a number of other chronic illness groups, including HIV+Stage 1, hemodialysis, long-term bone marrow transplant, liver transplant, dialysis, post angioplasty, coronary artery disease, post chemotherapy cancer, spouses of coronary bypass, and narcolepsy (Anderson & Ferrans, 1997). The current U.S. definition (Fukuda et al., 1994) requires that the following criteria be met for the diagnosis of CFS to be made: (a) 6 or more months of persistent or relapsing chronic fatigue of new or definite onset that is neither the result of ongoing exertion nor alleviated by rest, and results in substantial reductions in previous levels of occupational, educational, social, or personal activities; and (b) the concurrent occurrence of four or more of eight minor symptoms that persist or reoccur during 6 or more months of the illness and do not predate the fatigue. These eight minor symptoms include impairment in short-term memory or concentration severe enough to cause substantial reductions in previous levels of occupational, educational, social, or personal activities; sore throat; tender cervical or axillary lymph nodes; muscle pain; multiple joint pain without joint swelling or redness; headaches of a new type, pattern, or severity; unrefreshing sleep; and postexertional malaise lasting more than 24 hours. This definition was based upon expert consensus and was not empirically derived. Therefore, it should be considered as preliminary, requiring further validation. Chronic fatigue syndrome has been recognized as a disability by Social Security, and confirmed as a legitimate clinical entity by the U.S. Centers for Disease Control and Prevention. Numerous results from biomedical studies have also confirmed its medical legitimacy and significance as a public health concern. Further discussion about diagnostic criteria for CFS is presented by Friedberg and Jason (1998).

Fibromyalgia (FMS) is also a common illness condition characterized by chronic, generalized muscle pain, particular sensitivity to pressure in specific areas of the body (known as "tender points"), fatigue, and disrupted sleep. It is also associated with myofascial pain syndrome, Candida infection, headache, irritable bowel syndrome, Crohn's disease, and interstitial cystitis; occurs most commonly in women; and may follow an acute medical illness, traumatic injury, or surgery (Waylonis & Perkins, 1994). Fibromyalgia is estimated to occur in approximately 2% of the population (Wolfe et al., 1995). About 3.4% of women and .5% of men within the U.S. meet criteria for FMS (Wolfe et al., 1995). Current criteria for the diagnosis of FMS require widespread muscular pain in conjunction with tenderness at a minimum number of tender points (11 of 18) (Wolfe et al., 1990). While empirically derived, this definition should be considered as preliminary and as requiring further validation. Fibromyalgia is recognized as an illness by the American College of Rheumatology, the American Medical Association, the World Health Organization, and the National Institutes of Health. Further discussion of diagnostic criteria for FMS, including questions and answers about common symptoms, is presented by Starlanyl and Copeland (1996).

Multiple chemical sensitivities (MCS) is a chronic condition of irritation or inflammation of sensory organs, gastrointestinal distress, fatigue, and compromised neurological function, including learning and memory deficits, hypersensitivity to unpleasant smells, tingling of nerves, and sensory discomfort. It is a condition in which individuals experience symptoms, often in multiple organ systems, when they come in contact with low level exposure to certain chemical agents. Onset usually occurs either as a result of a high-level toxic chemical exposure (usually volatile, odoriferous solvents, pesticides, or exposures such as auto exhaust or smoke) or as a result of prolonged exposure to low-levels of toxicity over a period of years. Following initial sensitization, symptoms are triggered by common exposures (referred to as "triggering") and increase in number and severity over time (referred to as "spreading"). Typical symptoms include those of skin and/or mucous membrane irritation (e.g., nasal stuffiness, shortness of breath), fatigue, myalgias, fevers, irritability, dizziness, and neurocognitive dysfunction (Davis, Jason, & Banghart, 1998). The most recent case definition of MCS describes it as a chronic condition in which symptoms recur reproducibly in response to low levels of exposure to multiple, unrelated chemicals. Symptoms must occur in multiple organ systems and can either improve or resolve when the incitants are removed (Bartha et al., 1999). This definition was based upon expert consensus and should be considered as preliminary and requiring further validation. Standardized use of these criteria in clinical settings is lacking and greatly needed, given the high estimated prevalence of this condition within the United States. (Further discussion of prior case definitions of MCS and of the history behind MCS diagnosis is presented in Ross et al., 1999.) Multiple chemical sensitivities is one of the most commonly diagnosed chronic disorders, with a recently completed telephone survey indicating that 6% of adults in California were diagnosed with MCS, and 16% of respondents reported that they were unusually sensitive to everyday chemicals (Kreutzer, Neutra, & Lashuay, 1999). State health department surveys of individuals living in New Mexico and California have demonstrated prevalence rates of between 2% to 6%, or between 2,000 and 6,000 per 100,000 individuals. Common chemicals that trigger reactions include pesticides, perfumes, and detergent residues (Donnay, 1998). Many individuals with MCS are also allergic to various foods and food chemicals. These individuals with food allergies commonly experience bowel dysfunction and respond positively to elimination of certain foods from their diet. In addition to food allergies, individuals with MCS often report heightened sensitivity to sound, light, heat, cold, or touch. While physicians are generally skeptical about the nature of MCS, it is recognized as a disorder by the American Lung Association, American

Medical Association, U.S. Environmental Protection Agency, and the U.S. Consumer Product Safety Commission.

Chronic exposure to carbon monoxide (CO) has been found to produce chronic symptoms that are similar to CFS, FMS, and MCS (Hay, Jaffer, & Davies, 2000). A controlled study (Hay et al., 2000) documented the following symptoms as most prevalent among individuals chronically exposed to carbon monoxide: muscle pain (87.7%), headaches (86.2%), tiredness/weakness (89.2%), nausea/sickness (84.6%), and lack of concentration/confusion (76.9%). Clinicians should be aware that symptom presentations resembling CFS, FMS, and MCS may have alternative medical explanations, such as carbon monoxide poisoning. Hay and associates (2000) found that a diagnosis of CO poisoning was made by a clinician in only 13% of a group chronically exposed, and in 5% of these cases a diagnosis was made only after the individual lost consciousness due to the exposure. Misdiagnoses made by clinicians before discovery of CO poisoning included: 57% no diagnosis; 15% flu/virus; 8.5% depression; 5% chronic fatigue syndrome; 3% asthma; 3% psychosomatic; and 8.5% other/not available (Hay et al., 2000).

Gulf War Syndrome (GWS) is a recently described illness that shares many characteristics of CFS, FMS, and MCS. Although we do not present an in-depth analysis of the illness in this book, a brief overview is provided in this section. Gulf War Syndrome is characterized by symptoms that appear to reflect a spectrum of neurologic injury involving the central, peripheral, and autonomic nervous systems (Haley, Kurt, & Hom, 1997). These include problems with attention, memory, thinking, and reasoning, as well as insomnia, depression, daytime sleepiness, headaches, disorientation, balance disturbances, vertigo, sexual dysfunction, muscle and joint pains, muscle fatigue, difficulty lifting, and extremity paresthesias (numbness) (Haley et al., 1997). Five years after the Persian Gulf War, clusters of these symptoms continued to be reported by an estimated 5,000 to 80,000 of the U.S. veterans involved in the 1991 Gulf war against Iraq (Haley et al., 1997). Despite significant medical skepticism about GWS phenomenology by some research groups, other researchers have attributed Gulf War Syndrome symptoms to pesticide exposure, drug and chemical weapons exposures, or treatable infections such as Leishmania tropica (sand fly fever) and Mycoplasma fermentans (incognitus—bacterial infection that produces symptomatology similar to GWS, CFS, and FMS) (Donnay, 1998; Haley & Kurt, 1997).

More information about Gulf War Syndrome can be obtained from the
National Gulf War Resource Center, 1224 M Street NW, Washington,
DC 20005; (202) 628-2700, ext. 162.

## Patient Stigmatization

Controversial illnesses are stigmatizing to the patients who have
them. Physicians may dismiss patients' complaints and refuse to offer
treatment. Physicians who dispute the existence of these illnesses may
believe that the specific diagnoses of CFS, FMS, or MCS promote
illness-maintaining behavior. Yet such disbelief is highly stressful to
these patients, who are already bewildered by symptoms that they do
not understand and cannot control. Generally, patients feel reassured
by the diagnosis, which both validates their symptoms and excludes
degenerative diseases with similar symptoms. In our view, accurate
diagnosis allows patients to concentrate on coping and improving to
whatever extent possible rather than continuing the search for a diagnosis, a specific cause, or a simple cure. While there is some indica-
tion of movement toward change within the medical community,
widespread medical condescension toward these illnesses has, in large
part, been uncritically accepted by the public, as well as by family and
friends who may also view individuals with these conditions with
skepticism and even ridicule. What is the basis of such pervasive
disbelief?

First, the absence of a biological marker or diagnostic test to identify these illnesses places them in a dubious medical category of
vaguely defined and poorly understood chronic conditions. To many
physicians, such illnesses may be considered psychiatric disorders,
cases of malingering, or simply nonentities that are unworthy of seri-
ous attention. Even mental health professionals may be skeptical — an
unfortunate fact given their clinical expertise in coping and stress
reduction interventions. For example, a CFS clinical workshop that we
taught at the 1997 meeting of the American Psychological Association filled to capacity with over 50 psychologists, yet the majority
of them expressed profound skepticism of CFS and seemed to believe
that it was a nonillness. Unfortunately, such biases will not only interfere with the clinician's ability to help these patients, these attitudes
may trigger iatrogenic stress due to the delegitimizing effects of reject-
ing patients' concerns.

Second, patients are disbelieved and potentially stigmatized
because of their outwardly healthy appearances. Fatigue, in particular,

is a symptom that is not associated with any behavioral sign. And people with FMS, despite severely painful symptoms, can be quite successful in hiding them and in "passing" for healthy. Individuals with MCS also may appear superficially healthy although their sensitivity to chemical exposures may require escape and avoidance techniques that may alert others to their illness. Generally, patients with controversial illnesses do not display obvious illness behavior (e.g., wheelchair travel, impaired gait) that health professionals or the public would associate with disability. Therefore, it is assumed that their illnesses, even if real, could not be that severe.

Third, the enormous variation in symptom severity that can allow patients to be relatively functional for brief intervals yet severely impaired at other times is very difficult for others to comprehend. Rather than viewing these fluctuations as a manifestation of a highly unpredictable and poorly understood condition, observers are more likely to believe that disability and functionality are voluntary choices made by the patient. Several years ago, a respected radio talk show physician, Dr. Dean Edell, surmised that people with CFS who were demonstrating for more recognition and research funding must want to be sick — after all, they had no identifiable medical illness. And could they really be sick if they had enough energy to protest? Unfortunately, such a cynical view of controversial illnesses is not uncommon. Some physicians make the odd assumption that we know all we need to know about these illnesses, thus obviating the need for further research and greater understanding of these patients.

Fourth, negative attitudes may, in part, be a function of past portrayals of these illnesses as either nonexistent or as expressions of a neurotic, overworked, stressed lifestyle, as was depicted in the popular media label for CFS, "Yuppie Flu." Such media images hold individuals responsible for their illness without consideration for the complex and disabling nature of these conditions. This phenomenon of victim-blaming is reflected in the fundamental attribution error known as "belief in a just world," the belief that life justly rewards or punishes people for their actions through good or bad fortune.

Finally, with respect to CFS, disbelief has been generated by the use of the term, chronic fatigue syndrome, to describe the illness. Patient advocacy groups contend that this name tends to minimize the seriousness and complexity of the illness, and recent research supports this argument (Jason, Taylor, S. Plioplys, et al., in press; Jason, Taylor, Stepanek, et al., in press). Findings from two studies have indicated that the name, chronic fatigue syndrome, may be regarded less seriously than the myalgic encephalopathy name with respect to some important aspects of the illness, including attributions regarding illness cause. The myalgic encephalopathy name was significantly more likely than the chronic fatigue syndrome name to prompt attributions for a medical cause rather than a psychiatric cause.

## Chapter Previews

Chapter 1 presents the current case definitions and prevalence estimates for CFS, FMS, and MCS and briefly discusses Gulf War Syndrome. In addition, challenges facing practitioners involved in the treatment of individuals with these conditions, including issues involving patient stigmatization, are presented. In Chapter 2, proposed causal factors are reviewed for each illness, and their potential for integration within a biopsychosocial model is discussed. The following chapter (Chapter 3) explains the complex issue of differential diagnosis in controversial illness and overlapping psychiatric disorders. Case examples are given to illustrate how differential diagnosis can be made. Chapter 4 provides a brief overview of pen-and-paper measures for fatigue, pain, depression, anxiety, and generalized distress. Equally important to the clinician is the discussion of *in vivo* assessments which can identify important relationships between stress, activity, pain, fatigue and other symptoms. Chapter 5 reviews pharmacological approaches as well as alternative treatments to controversial illnesses. Chapter 6, Cognitive-Behavioral Treatment I, explores envelope theory as a method of activity management. Chapter 7, Cognitive-Behavioral Treatment II, focuses on coping skills techniques, particularly those derived from cognitive therapy and relaxation training. Brief case studies of these interventions illustrate how these techniques may be incorporated into clinical protocols. Chapter 8 offers future directions for clinicians and researchers.

Finally, the Appendices include useful diagnostic measures designed to screen for CFS, FMS, and MCS, and other rating scales that can assist clinicians in evaluating behavioral functioning, illness-related attitudes and beliefs, and psychosocial phases of development. The Chronic Fatigue Syndrome Self-Report Questionnaire in Appendix A (pp. 97–103) is a brief, in-office screening scale designed for use by clinicians to evaluate symptoms of the current U.S. criteria for CFS (Fukuda et al., 1994). The CFS Screening Questionnaire, presented in Appendix B (pp. 105–128) is a more comprehensive scale designed not only to measure symptoms of CFS, FMS, and MCS but also to evaluate patient history, medical exclusionary illnesses, and other potential medical and psychological contributors to fatigue. Appendices C to F (pp. 129–140) contain psychosocial and psychological tools measuring attitudes, behaviors, and cognitions associated with fatigue-related conditions that may be used during various phases of treatment. Appendix G (pp. 141–145) contains a list of useful resources for clinicians and patients with these conditions.

# CHAPTER 2

# Etiology and Perpetuating Factors

## Chronic Fatigue Syndrome

### Overview

CFS-like illnesses have been described in the medical literature since the mid-19th century and have carried names such as neurasthenia, brucellosis, Royal free disease, Iceland disease, and postviral fatigue. With the rediscovery of chronic fatigue syndrome in the 1980s, some theoreticians explained the flu-like symptoms of the illness as a chronic virus or an abnormality of the immune system. More recently, genetic factors have been implicated in twin studies of CFS patients. Debate regarding the medical legitimacy of CFS has entered into a number of important domains involving assessment and treatment for individuals with this syndrome. Some emphasize the role of psychological agents in the etiology and course of CFS and consider most patients presenting with CFS as having a form of somatic depression, conversion disorder, somatic anxiety, or some other variant of somatoform disorder. Others underscore the role of social-environmental factors in CFS, employing models of a dialectical relationship between body and society, in which somatic symptoms are interpreted as a consequence of painful or otherwise exploitative social interactions. Research applying this model (alternatively referred to as the "psychosocial model") suggests that, prior to becoming ill, individuals with CFS led overextended lifestyles, were exposed to high numbers of pre-illness stressful events, and received low levels of social support. However, more recent research contradicts some aspects of this model, finding no evidence for an association between fatigue, mood, and perfectionism (Blenkiron, Edwards, & Lynch, 1999). (More information about the psychosocial and psychiatric models is presented in the book *Understanding Chronic Fatigue Syndrome: An Empirical Guide to Assessment and Treatment* by Fred Friedberg & Leonard A. Jason, 1998.) Yet others emphasize the biomedical correlates of CFS, highlighting distinctions between CFS and psychiatric disorders such as depression (Lapp, 1992). Despite this controversy, a majority of researchers and practitioners now acknowledge some distinction between CFS and psychiatric illness or support a biopsychosocial model for understanding the etiology and course of CFS (Friedberg & Jason, 1998). This chapter will emphasize current biological and biopsychosocial explanations of CFS, acknowledging that few well-designed studies have been conducted to test these models.

## Biological Findings

Pathophysiological findings in microbiology, immunology, endocrinology, and neurology-related fields suggest that CFS cannot be explained by psychiatric factors alone, and laboratory studies have detected differences between individuals with CFS and those with primary depression on a number of indices (DeLuca et al., 1997; Demitrack et al., 1991; S. Plioplys & A. V. Plioplys, 1995; Suhadolnik, Reichenbach, Hitzges, Adelson, et al., 1994). For example, Demitrack and associates (1991) detected lower basal cortisol (stress hormone) levels and higher basal adrenocorticotropic hormone (ACTH) in a sample of individuals with CFS, a pattern opposite to the basal hypercortisolism and normal levels of ACTH typically found in patients with primary depression. Similarly, a randomized, double-blind, placebo-controlled study of the effects of fluoxetine (antidepressant Prozac) in CFS found that a 20 mg per day dosage had no beneficial effect on any of the CFS symptoms (Vercoulen et al., 1996). Using single-photon emission computed tomography (SPECT) procedures, Schwartz and associates (1994) found neurophysiological evidence suggesting that chronic fatigue syndrome may be due to a chronic viral encephalitis. These researchers compared neurological abnormalities in patients with CFS, AIDS dementia complex, major unipolar depression, and healthy controls, and found that the midcerebral uptake index (reflecting different patterns of blood flow to this area of the brain) was significantly lower in the CFS and AIDS dementia complex patients as compared with those with major depression or healthy controls. Also, the number of regional defects was significantly correlated with the midcerebral uptake index in those with CFS and AIDS dementia complex but not in depressed patients or controls. Results such as these suggest that there are different neurochemical processes underlying the presence of depressive-type symptoms in CFS and major depression.

Another study comparing functional impairment in participants with CFS, hypertension, congestive heart failure, diabetes, multiple sclerosis, acute myocardial infarction, and depression found highest levels of physical impairment in CFS patients on virtually all measures (Komaroff et al., 1996). Contrary to the depressive patients, participants with CFS showed greater impairment in overall health and work due to physical health problems, but less mental health impairment (Komaroff et al., 1996). Moreover, almost every investigation of psychiatric comorbidity conducted to date has found an absence of diagnosable psychiatric illness in at least one-quarter to one-third of individuals with CFS (Wessely, 1998). Findings such as these support the medical legitimacy of CFS.

## Explanatory Models of CFS

*Immune Activation Model*

The immune activation model is one biological explanation positing that CFS and its associated allergies and neuropsychiatric symptoms are triggered by a persistent overactivation of the immune system, which produces flu-like symptoms. Such flu-like symptoms include sore throat, lymph node pain, fatigue, headache, muscle pain, sleep disturbance, and temperature dysregulation. These symptoms are normally associated with transitory acute illnesses and then disappear once the pathogenic agent has been subdued by immune defenses. According to the model, however, the immune response remains elevated despite the absence of an identified invading pathogen. Evidence for chronic immune activation in subsets of individuals with CFS includes elevations in activated T lymphocytes and poor cellular function as represented by natural killer cell cytotoxicity and frequent immunoglobulin deficiencies (most often IgG1 and IgG3), reduced suppressor cell population in conjunction with elevated immune activation markers (CD38 and HLA-DR), deficits in cortisol and corticotropin-releasing hormone, and increased levels of adhesion markers in memory T cells (Friedberg & Jason, 1998).

*Sleep Disorder Model*

Recently, Hickie and Davenport (1999) proposed that, regardless of original etiology, most cases of CFS are best viewed as chronic disorders of the sleep-wake cycle. According to these researchers, a range of physical and psychological disorders, including CFS, may result in a preferential reduction of deep (stages three and four or slow-wave) sleep that alters overall sleep architecture and neurohormonal cycles (i.e., circadian rhythms). CFS is hence described as a "zombie-like" state from both neurohormonal and symptomatic perspectives. On a symptomatic level, individuals with CFS report that they have great difficulty remaining alert and awake during the day but also have great difficulty switching over to deep sleep at night. Thus, they feel "half-asleep" during both the day and night. From a neurohormonal perspective, most have lost their circadian rhythms or moved out of synchrony with regular environmental cues, such as sunrise and sunset. As a result, they no longer possess the neurohormonal substrate for either normal wakefulness (high cortisol, increased body temperature, low melatonin) or normal restorative sleep (high melatonin, low cortisol, low body temperature). According to this model, patient reports of morning fatigue, unrefreshing sleep, and nausea are, in fact, responding appropriately to their actual neurohormonal state (lack of slow-wave sleep and low, rather than rising cortisol levels). Thus, the key to successful behavioral interventions according to Hickie and Davenport (1999) is for individuals to engage in physical and environmental activities that may serve to "reset" the natural biological and hormonal clock.

## Explanatory Models of Fibromyalgia

Similar to explanatory models for CFS, there are currently no identifiable etiological agents explaining the onset and chronicity of FMS symptoms. The models of FMS (Ang & Wilkes, 1999) presented herein have widely varying levels of theoretical development and evidentiary support. No consensus on the validity of any of these models has been reached. While the following section focuses primarily on biologic and behavioral factors that may be linked to either the cause or perpetuation of FMS, it is not exhaustive of extant theories on this topic. It is likely that multiple interacting factors, including neurohormonal and psychological influences, may eventually lead to an integrated biopsychosocial model of the illness.

## Sleep Disturbance

A primary sleep disturbance has been proposed as a putative causal factor in fibromyalgia. Patient-reported sleep disturbance is ubiquitous in the illness, and consistent evidence has been reported for a loss of stage four (slow-wave) non-REM sleep in fibromyalgia patients. Research has found that healthy individuals who are deprived of stage four sleep also develop an FMS-like syndrome. It has been suggested that abnormal serotonin metabolism (which is important in the regulation of deep sleep and pain) and elevated levels of substance P (a mediator of pain reception) may be the basis of sleep disturbance in FMS. On a behavioral level, sleep disturbance can be activated by physical overexertion, emotional stress, postural abnormalities, use of alcohol or caffeine (particularly within a few hours before bedtime), menopausal hot flashes, or environmental disruptions (e.g., noise).

## Infectious Agents

As in CFS, infectious agents that produce flu-like symptoms have also been explored as a causal factor in FMS. Suspected agents have included Epstein-Barr virus, cytomegalovirus, and enteroviruses. Although many of these agents have been ruled out as causative factors, it is thought by some researchers that such infections may lead susceptible people into a compromised immune state which produces FMS symptoms.

## Neuroendocrine Abnormalities

The neuroendocrine axes are essential physiologic systems that allow for communication between the brain and the body. The hypothalamic-pituitary-adrenal (HPA) axis plays a pivotal role in the coordinated physiologic response to physical and emotional stress. Individuals with FMS tend to show physiologic hyperarousal in their pattern of HPA axis response. This persistent exaggerated activity of the HPA is postulated by some theoreticians as an important factor in the onset and maintenance of the symptom complex in FMS. This model has also been applied in understanding CFS.

## Explanatory Models of Multiple Chemical Sensitivities

Despite an abundance of theories about the origins of MCS (Weiss, 1997), clear evidence for any explanatory model is lacking. This lack of understanding is in part due to the paucity of research on the illness. Some of the more well-known and recent theoretical models are presented in the following sections.

### Time-Dependent Sensitization and Limbic Kindling

The kindling hypothesis (Bell et al., 1997) proposes that changes in brain function could lead to MCS. Kindling provides a neurophysiological explanation for observations of spreading aversions and central nervous system involvement in individuals with MCS. According to the kindling hypothesis — which follows a pattern known as time-dependent sensitization — intermittent, repeated, low-level odorant exposures are proposed to cause a sensitized state in the limbic system of the brain, which is involved in regulating emotions such as anxiety and depression. This sensitized state would subsequently amplify the response to low-level odors, initiating persistent affective, cognitive, and somatic symptomatology that increase over time. Hypothesized factors contributing to this susceptibility may include genetic factors, shyness, early life trauma, toxic exposures, and kindling in the classic sense of repeated, low-level stressors (Ross et al., 1999).

As noted by Ross and associates (1999), some features of MCS are difficult to explain within a limbic kindling framework. For example, repeated, unrecognized exposures that provoke neural after-discharges are required for kindling, and this contradicts most MCS case definitions as well as patient reports, which indicate an initial, and often single, sensitizing type of exposure to a high-level of toxicity. Similarly, Miller (1992) points out that, while it is plausible that thought processes and mood states may trigger or interrupt preexisting limbic activity, no evidence suggests that limbic activity triggered by environmental exposures can be entirely treated by psychological interventions.

### Allergy or Immune System Dysregulation

Some studies have linked MCS to allergy or immune system dysregulation, positing that MCS is a disease that spreads between various target organs and is caused by sensitization to chemicals with very different structures. In the case of allergies, MCS has been known to elicit bronchial symptoms similar to those observed in asthma and reactive airway dysfunction syndrome. Under the immune system dysregulation model, MCS is attributed to free radical production and stress, which indirectly cause spreading because of damage to the immune system. In other words, MCS results from toxicity to the immune system, and some investigators have reported subtle alterations in certain aspects of immune function or cell counts. However, these findings have not been replicated on a large-scale basis, and case controlled studies have found no evidence that individuals with MCS have compromised immune symptoms. In part, this absence of findings may be attributable to the fact that one of the earlier, widely used definitions of MCS (Cullen, 1987) specifically excluded patients with verifiable signs of toxicity syndromes. In conclusion, Ross and associates (1999) suggest that the evidence does not support the view that MCS is like known immunotoxic phenomena and that MCS may be only peripherally related to immune sensitization. Thus, Ross and associates refute this model and contend that it is unlikely that fragrances can produce MCS symptoms through allergic mechanisms.

**Neurotoxicity Model**

Some researchers argue that MCS may result from the introduction of a toxic chemical directly into the brain through the olfactory epithelium, with the assumption that substances most commonly implicated in the development of MCS (pesticides and solvents) are neurotoxic at some level. This model is based on evidence for short-term memory deficit, cognitive depression, and cacosmia among individuals with MCS. This model posits that MCS is different from neurotoxicity in the traditional sense because MCS symptoms are transitory and there are no widely accepted objective signs in MCS. Unlike individuals with MCS, solvent-poisoned patients with measurable forms of neurotoxicity exhibit measurable brain pathology and do not report cyclical symptom episodes in response to subsequent exposures. According to this model, however, it is possible that individuals with MCS may characterize the lowest grade of solvent neurotoxicity (Type 1), which may be reversible upon removal from the agent and may not be associated with objective evidence of impairment, or they may more commonly characterize the next highest category of neurotoxicity (Type 2a), in which symptoms may or may not be reversible upon removal from the agent but remain undetectable according to measures of brain damage upon neuropsychologic examination. Like the other models, this model is preliminary and not uniformly supported in the research.

### Upper Airway Irritancy

A group of investigators has proposed that MCS symptoms result from chronic, upper airway inflammation, sinusitis, or neurogenic inflammation. Associations between upper airway inflammation and MCS symptoms are consistent with general observations of links between environmental air quality deterioration and MCS outbreaks. Some propose that individuals with MCS have been sensitized through time spent in "sick" buildings, which contained air irritants that ultimately led to upper airway pathology. Under this hypothesis, both MCS and "sick building syndrome" are considered as resulting from altered responsiveness of C-fiber neurons in the upper respiratory mucosa and an amplification of a nonspecific immune response to low level irritants in the upper airways. Like the other models, this model is preliminary and requires further research for validation.

### Clinical Ecology

A conceptualization of MCS based on the principles of clinical ecology suggests that an accumulation of physical and emotional stressors will adversely affect vulnerable individuals. These assaults to the body will lead to "exhaustion" of biological defenses and illness formation. These illness-producing stressors include exposure to toxic chemicals in the air, food, and water, as well as to emotional stress. The proposed breakdown of the body's defensive mechanisms allows the takeover by viruses, bacteria, or other infectious agents. Despite its popularity among some clinical physicians and patient groups, this model lacks empirical support.

## Models Addressing Psychosocial Aspects of CFS, FMS, and MCS

As with biological models, models addressing psychosocial aspects of these controversial illnesses have not been supported consistently in the research. Models addressing psychosocial aspects of CFS, FMS, and MCS offer potentially useful constructs for the clinician in formulating assessment and treatment strategies. While we believe that theories of pure psychogenesis represent an oversimplification of the biopsychosocial complexities of these conditions, we can acknowledge a role for psychological and behavioral factors without negating the reality of these debilitating conditions. Even for those individuals with controversial illnesses who do not have concurrent psychiatric disorders, psychological and stress factors do play important roles in the illness experience. Presented on the following pages are examples of such models in order to allow for better understanding of the role of psychological variables in these conditions, particularly for patients with prominent psychiatric overlays more commonly encountered in psychotherapy practice.

**Illness Reactivity Model**

The illness reactivity model (Friedberg & Jason, 1998) postulates that a combination of predisposing biological factors and health-damaging behaviors trigger illnesses such as chronic fatigue syndrome. The stress generated by these health-damaging behaviors propels the vulnerable individual into partial exhaustion states, which eventuate in chronic fatigue syndrome. Then, psychological reactions to the illness and its limitations (including depression, anxiety, and anger) engender increased fatigue which, in turn, exacerbates symptoms. These emotional reactions are triggered by understandably negative thoughts about the illness and its impact on the affected individual's vocational, interpersonal, and recreational activities.

A coping skills-oriented cognitive behavioral intervention can teach the patient to interrupt the cycle of symptom-exacerbating stress (Friedberg, 1996). Improved coping skills will reduce symptoms of depression, anxiety, and anger. In patients with CFS who attempt to maintain damaging pre-illness behaviors, healthy modifications of these patterns, such as overwork and unhealthy dependency, may result in significant illness improvements. In other patients who remain disabled with the illness, despite lifestyle modifications, illness-coping strategies that minimize stress and generate optimism may be most appropriate. The illness reactivity model has received initial empirical support from a coping skills treatment study (Friedberg & Krupp, 1994).

**Models Focusing on Personality Factors**

*"Pain Prone Personality"*

A stressful hyperactive lifestyle prior to illness onset has also been proposed as an important element in the development of FMS. One theory invokes the so-called "pain prone" personality (Blumer &

Heilbronn, 1981) as an important precursor of FMS. The "pain prone" personality shows an extreme orientation toward high achievement and perfectionism combined with an inability to relax and enjoy leisure. Associated traits include altruism linked with a lack of assertiveness; denial of emotional and interpersonal conflicts; excessive dependency; and an inability to perceive and express unpleasant feelings like anger, frustration, and sadness (i.e., alexithymia). This excessive striving for achievement coupled with assertiveness deficits may be responsible for persistently elevated levels of stress which may lead to FMS in susceptible individuals. The core element of these personality traits seems to be an unstable self-esteem that depends excessively on the acceptance and recognition by others through high achievement. According to this model, adverse childhood experiences like poverty, lack of affection, repetitive trauma, or physical and sexual abuse may also increase susceptibility to FMS. Although this model was originally conceived as a comprehensive psychodynamic theory of many chronic pain conditions, we view it, in light of modern behavioral medicine theory, as one possible predisposing factor in FMS, rather than as a simple cause-effect explanation. A comparative study of individuals with FMS and those with other conditions involving chronic pain (Amir et al., 2000) did not find significant differences in coping styles and trait anger between illness groups. Anger and avoidance coping were significantly higher in all of the illness groups as compared with the healthy control group (Amir et al., 2000).

*Phobic Avoidance/Conditioning Model*

The phobic avoidance/conditioning model of MCS (Guglielmi, Cox, & Spyker, 1994) proposes that chemical sensitivities in MCS patients are an atypical type of phobic disturbance in which neutral, often olfactory stimuli can come to produce panic symptoms as conditioned responses. Stimulus generalization is commonly seen in this type of learning, leading to increased anticipatory anxiety and phobic avoidance of perceived triggers. This reaction can produce an ever-shrinking sphere of comfortable living space for the patient. The panic attacks are mistakenly believed to be produced by the odor itself (conditioned stimulus) in the environment. Treatment consists of behavioral desensitization involving graded exposure to phobic stimuli and pharmacological control of hyperarousal and panic (see Chapter 7).

*Symptom Avoidance Model*

The symptom avoidance model (Surawy et al., 1995) proposes that an initial acute illness combined with severe psychosocial stress triggers CFS symptoms. As the acute illness subsides, disability persists due to the patient's fear of increasing symptoms through exertion and activity. Thus, a cycle of fear-based behavioral avoidance maintains CFS symptoms which in turn produces demoralization and further distress. Controlled clinical trials (e.g., Deale et al., 1997) conducted in England of graded activity schedules in combination with cognitive restructuring of irrational fears of symptom flare-ups have reportedly reversed the disabling effects and chronic symptoms of the illness.

Although these clinical trials appear to impressively demonstrate the efficacy of graded activity-oriented cognitive-behavioral therapy, it is possible that the patients selected for these trials include a phobic-like subset of CFS patients that may not be representative of the CFS population generally (Friedberg, 1999). In CFS patients without fear-based avoidance, or for patients who are already performing at their maximum activity levels, it is not clear that graded activity intervention will produce such favorable outcomes.

## Biopsychosocial and Psychoneuroimmunological Models: A Unifying Approach to Understanding CFS, FMS, and MCS

The biopsychosocial model (Friedberg & Jason, 1998) contends that there might be multiple pathways leading to the cause and maintenance of the neurobiologic disregulations and other symptoms experienced by individuals with CFS, FMS, and MCS. Depending upon the individual, these may include unique biological, genetic, neurological, psychological, and socioenvironmental contributions. One strength of a biopsychosocial understanding of CFS, FMS, and MCS is that it may serve as a means of bridging the theoretical gap between mind versus body explanations of these illnesses. Similarly, a psychoneuroimmunological model (Jason et al., 1995) can provide another comprehensive heuristic framework for understanding these complex illnesses. Psychoneuroimmunology presents an alternative to current research-induced dichotomous conceptualizations as solely diseases of the body or the mind. A psychoneuroimmunological model suggests that an ongoing connection exists between nervous, endocrine, and immune systems within the body. Consequently, conditions of stress, depression, anxiety, loss of control, learned helplessness, high anxiety, loneliness, bereavement, or high inhibited power motivation may interfere with adequate immune functioning. Psychological and environmental factors may serve to influence immunosuppression, including dysphoric responses (e.g., depressive affect, unhappiness, anxiety), immunosuppressive behaviors (e.g., dietary patterns, sleep habits, licit and illicit drug use), adverse life experiences (e.g., ongoing strains in interpersonal relationships), and preexisting vulnerabilities (e.g., the absence of interpersonal resources and coping patterns to forestall the impact of negative life experiences). In summary, psychoneuroimmunology provides a transactional model, which accounts for complex interactions between multiple biological and psychological factors that influence both the onset of these syndromes and pathways to further illness or recovery. Despite the theoretical appeal of the biopsychosocial and psychoneuroimmunological models, recent twin studies of complex genetic and environmental relationships between psychological distress, fatigue, and immune system functioning suggest that these models need to acknowledge the increasing importance of the individual's genotype (Hickie et al., 1999).

# CHAPTER 3

# Diagnostic Issues

Many of the symptoms associated with CFS are also characteristic of other poorly understood illness conditions including fibromyalgia (FMS) and multiple chemical sensitivities (MCS). In the absence of definitive diagnostic markers or laboratory tests to distinguish these conditions, clinical diagnosis is largely based on self-report symptoms and behavioral criteria. The considerable overlap of symptoms experienced by people with CFS, FMS, and MCS has led some researchers to question whether diagnostic criteria for these conditions are able to adequately distinguish between the disorders as well as distinguish the conditions from psychiatric disorders involving components of somatization. Despite these speculations, however, many researchers and clinicians view these syndromes as distinct diagnostic entities.

One factor that has complicated the understanding of CFS is the lack of consensus among health care professionals regarding the interpretation and application of the diagnostic criteria. Since its emergence as a new disease category in the 1980s, four widely used definitions of CFS have been proposed through expert consensus (Fukuda et al., 1994; Holmes et al., 1988; Lloyd et al., 1990; Sharpe et al., 1991); none has been derived empirically. Perhaps as a result, clinicians and health care professionals working with chronically fatigued clients have noted a number of difficulties with each of these case definitions. For example, symptoms of sore throat or lymph node pain can only be confirmed infrequently by a physician, and other symptomatic criteria are even more difficult to confirm because of their ambiguous nature (e.g., difficulty concentrating). Additional challenges faced by those who attempt to define CFS include (Friedberg & Jason, 1998; Jason, King, et al., 1999):

1. *Balancing sensitivity and specificity in diagnosis.* Criteria that is too general may fail to adequately exclude people who have alternative explanations for their fatigue, such as primary psychiatric disorders, stress, or psychosocial explanations. Overly strict criteria may inappropriately exclude someone from a diagnosis.

2. *Accounting for patient heterogeneity.* Research has suggested that individuals with CFS can be subtyped along a number of indices, including mode of onset. For example, Johnson, DeLuca, and Natelson (1999) suggest that there might be two groups of individuals with CFS; one with sudden illness onset, no psychiatric comorbidity, and serious cognitive impairment; and another with slow onset, psychiatric comorbidity, and mild cognitive impairment. Because CFS tends to fluctuate in terms of symptoms and severity, health care professionals must be careful to assess all areas of functioning (e.g., occupational, educational, social, and personal activities) across a reliable period of time. For some individuals with CFS, it is possible to work full-time during certain phases of the illness at the expense of social or personal activities. Case criteria should accommodate such issues of patient heterogeneity through subtyping.

In sum, defining CFS is fraught with pragmatic and theoretical difficulties. In response to a need to develop objective clinical means of distinguishing individuals with CFS from those with other illnesses, Caroline King, Dr. Leonard Jason, and Dr. Renée Taylor from DePaul University have developed a brief self-report questionnaire modeled after the current Centers for Disease Control (CDC) case definition (Fukuda et al., 1994), which incorporates additional empirical findings for symptom patterns in individuals with CFS. This brief questionnaire, presented in Appendix A (pp. 97–103), can be useful to the mental health clinician in assessing the primary symptomatology and impairments associated with CFS.

While inconclusive, the following represents a list of additional biological issues to think about in assessing individuals with CFS (Verrillo & Gellman, 1997). Depending upon the patient, these issues may be more or less relevant to understanding symptomatology, but researchers have identified some of these issues as possible directions for future investigation and understanding. These include:

1. positive viral laboratory findings for Epstein-Barr virus, human herpesvirus 6, coxsackievirus, cytomegalovirus, and negative findings for hepatitis A or B virus;
2. immunological findings revealing low natural killer cell counts, elevated interferon alpha, tumor necrosis factor, interleukins 1 and 2, T cell activation, altered T4/T8 cell ratios, low T cell suppressor cell (T8) count, fluctuating low and high T cell counts, low and high B cell counts, antinuclear antibodies, immunoglobulin deficiency, and occasionally antithyroid antibodies;
3. abnormalities occurring after exercise, including muscle cell abnormalities, decreased cognitive functioning, decreased cortisol levels, decreased cerebral blood flow, inefficient glucose utilization, and erratic breathing pattern; and
4. SPECT scan findings for hypoperfusion in either right or left temporal lobes, particularly following exercise.

Other physical signs that have been noted in CFS upon physical examination include orthostatic hypotension; low (97° F) or slightly high (≤ 100° F) temperature, or both occurring over the course of the day (excessive diurnal variation); tachycardia detectable using Holter monitor; irritated, reddened throat; tender, palpable lymph nodes, particularly in groin and neck and on the left side of the body; persistent, reproducible muscle tenderness on repeated examinations; pallor of skin; positive Rhomberg test (tandem stance); and stiff, slow gait. Clinicians should note that the absence of these physical signs does not preclude a diagnosis of CFS.

Fibromyalgia syndrome and multiple chemical sensitivities are of additional interest where issues of diagnostic accuracy are concerned. Reports of high levels of reactivity to chemical exposures are common among individuals with CFS (Friedberg et al., 2000). A study by Buchwald and Garrity (1994) found that a majority of both CFS and FMS cohorts also experienced MCS and that the overlap between individuals with CFS and FMS was even higher. Donnay and Ziem (1998) reported on the prevalence and overlap of CFS and FMS among 100 patients with MCS. Of the 100 patients with MCS, 88% met the criteria for CFS. In a recent community-based study of 32 individuals with CFS (Jason, Taylor, & Kennedy, 2000), 40.6% met criteria for MCS, and 15.6% met criteria for FMS. Individuals with MCS or more than one diagnosis reported more physical fatigue than those with no diagnosis. Individuals with more than one diagnosis also reported greater mental fatigue and were less likely to be working than those with no diagnosis. Individuals with CFS, MCS, FMS, or more than one diagnosis reported greater disability than those with no diagnosis. Evaluating the presence of these three illnesses seems essential, particularly since it is probable that those individuals with CFS who are most ill have additional diagnoses of FMS and/or MCS.

Fibromyalgia was officially recognized as a syndrome on January 1, 1993 by the World Health Organization as a result of the Copenhagen Declaration (Consensus Document on Fibromyalgia: The Copenhagen Declaration, 1992). The Copenhagen Declaration defined FMS as a painful condition primarily involving muscles and not joints and as the most common cause of chronic, widespread musculoskeletal pain. One means of distinguishing FMS from CFS and MCS is by applying diagnostic criteria that was developed empirically (Wolfe et al., 1990) by the American College of Rheumatology and thus presumed to offer increased diagnostic validity. Wolfe and associates (1990) studied 558 consecutive patients: 293 with FMS and 265 controls. In terms of diagnostic criteria, they found that the combination of widespread pain and mild or greater tenderness in 11 or more of 18 tender point sites yielded a sensitivity of 88.4% and a specificity of 81.1%, indicating strong support for these diagnostic criteria. While nonrefreshing sleep, persistent fatigue, and generalized morning stiffness were central symptoms of FMS, with each present in more than 75% of patients, only 56% of patients had all three symptoms, so the simultaneous presence of these three symptoms was not required for a diagnosis of FMS. This study used standardized questionnaires to obtain historical information, collecting data that were free from interviewer-introduced bias (the examiners were not aware of the diagnosis or physical findings of the examination).

Tender points are painful when pressed (clinical anecdote suggests that the pressure required to produce pain is typically no greater than just enough to whiten the thumbnail). Distinct from the Wolfe et al. (1990) criteria, the Copenhagen definition of FMS also asserts a requirement that tender points must be present in all four quadrants of the body (i.e., above and below the waist on the right and left sides). In addition, widespread muscular pain must be present for at least 3 months. Because tender points tend to occur in pairs, the pain is usually present on both sides of the body. Although tender point location can vary from person to person, tender points are typically located

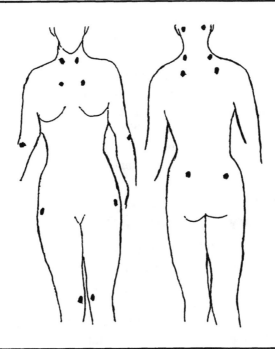

**Figure 1. Tender Point Locations.**

in 18 specific places, 10 on the front and 8 along the back of the body (see Figure 1 above).

One study indicated that there are additional clinical signs, apart from the tender points, which are abnormal in FMS and appear to be useful as objective signs in the assessment of these patients (Granges & Littlejohn, 1993). These included pain threshold to pressure, skinfold tenderness, and reactive skin hyperemia to pressure as significantly higher than for controls; and tissue compliance at trapezius, thoracic, and lumbar locations as significantly lower than for controls.

Multiple chemical sensitivities can best be differentiated from CFS and FMS due to the reactive nature of the illness upon exposure to relatively low levels of chemicals and other irritants, and the resolution of symptoms upon withdrawal from the chemicals or irritants. In addition, there are clinical reports of measurable signs of chemical reactivity and inhalation toxicity upon physical examination. These can include increased nasal resistance, upper airway inflammation, Positron Emission Tomography (PET) abnormalities reminiscent of pesticide-poisoned patients, and changes in chemosensory evoked potentials

(Ross et al., 1999), but they are not always replicated across studies. As is often the case, this distinction becomes less clear when individuals with CFS or FMS also suffer from chemical or food sensitivities, or from full-blown MCS. Some of the symptoms produced by the chemical exposure may also be a part of CFS or MCS (e.g., fatigue, cognitive dysfunction, dizziness, myalgias) and may not dissipate upon removal of the irritant. In these cases, MCS is best identified through careful observation of overall symptom exacerbation with exposures and overall symptom improvement with irritant removal.

## Differential Diagnoses: CFS, FMS, MCS Versus Primary Psychiatric Disorders

CFS, FMS, and MCS may share many symptoms with nonmelancholic depression, anxiety disorders, and somatoform disorders. Depending upon the condition and patient, overlapping symptoms may include fatigue, psychomotor retardation, difficulty concentrating, weight change, and sleep disturbance. Due to symptom overlap, superficial characterizations of these conditions may appear no different than those of many psychiatric disorders with primarily somatic manifestations. However, when one examines the symptoms, diagnostic criteria, and psychosocial context for each of these illnesses more carefully, important distinctions do arise. For example, one key distinguishing feature of CFS, as compared with psychiatric disorders, is exercise intolerance. Attempts to increase endurance and reduce symptoms through physical exercise often result in symptom flare-ups rather than physical improvements. In contrast, exercise programs, such as walking schedules, may be effective therapy for depressive and anxiety disorders. In addition, researchers have noted the following qualitative differences in CFS-related fatigue, including subjective ratings of fatigue as more severe and unusual sensations of fatigue similar to those found in a variety of medical conditions (Friedberg & Jason, 1998). Descriptions of this fatigue include arms or legs feeling "heavy" or "dead" at rest; difficulty with physical activity (e.g., climbing stairs described as "swimming against a current of molasses"); feeling as if "hit by a truck"; and having to consciously think about a movement and concentrate before completing it (Friedberg & Jason, 1998). Table 1 (p. 31) lists some of these distinctions measured by Komaroff and associates (1996).

Similar to the case of depression, the symptoms of somatoform disorders demonstrate considerable overlap with CFS. For example,

## Table 1: A Comparison of Reported Symptoms of Patients With CFS Versus Primary Depression*

| Symptoms | CFS | Depression |
|---|---|---|
| Severe Debilitating Fatigue | 100% | 28% |
| Acute Onset of Illness | 84% | 0% |
| Postexertional Malaise | 79%-87% | 19% |
| Alcohol Intolerance | 60% | 21% |
| Difficulty Falling Asleep | 53% | 26% |
| Early Morning Awakenings | 19% | 58% |
| Nausea | 58% | 16% |
| Flu-Like Symptoms (sore throat, painful lymph nodes, mild fevers, headaches) | 43%-65% | 10%-22% |
| Difficulty Concentrating | 83% | 79% |
| Loss of Sexual Desire | 54% | 58% |
| Joint Pain | 53% | 50% |

*Reprinted from *American Journal of Medicine*, Volume 100, Komaroff et al., "An Examination of the Working Case Definition of Chronic Fatigue Syndrome," pp. 56-64, 1996, with permission from Excerpta Medica, Inc.

the *DSM-IV* (American Psychiatric Association [APA], 1994) criteria for somatization disorder require four pain symptoms, two gastrointestinal symptoms, one sexual symptom, and one pseudoneurological symptom (e.g., impaired coordination or balance, paralysis or localized weakness, etc.). Though not all of these symptoms are listed as formal diagnostic criteria under the current definition (Fukuda et al., 1994), individuals with CFS may also present with gastrointestinal, pain, sexual, and neurological symptoms. Because neither condition can be fully explained medically and no diagnostic or laboratory tests are available to distinguish the two disorders, clinicians must be highly familiar with subtle differences in symptom presentation and illness context between the two disorders. Similar to the distinctions between CFS and depression noted by Komaroff and associates (1996), Friedberg and Jason (1998) observed a number of important differences between CFS and somatization disorder. First, while fatigue is the primary feature of CFS, this symptom is not a listed criterion of somatization disorder. Also, individuals with CFS typically report a sudden onset of the symptom complex, with the majority becoming ill after the age of 30, whereas initial symptoms of somatization disorder begin in adolescence, escalate over several years, and become full-blown somatization disorder by the age of 25 (APA, 1994). In addition, the patterning of somatization disorder symptoms can vary from person to person and does not often fit a distinctive profile, whereas the patterning of CFS is more consistent between different individuals with the disorder. Thus, in evaluating distinctions between the two disorders, one should assess the presence of multiple somatization symptoms prior to CFS onset, occurring in the absence of profound, debilitating fatigue.

Symptoms of CFS also overlap with symptoms of anxiety disorders. Friedberg and Jason (1998) noted that CFS and generalized anxiety disorder share the following symptoms in common: fatigue, difficulty concentrating, sleep disturbance, irritability, restlessness, and rapid heartbeat. The primary feature of generalized anxiety disorder is excessive, persistent worry, with the likelihood of diagnosis increasing as the individual worries about more and more life circumstances (e.g., finances, job performance, parenting issues) (APA, 1994). Given that individuals with CFS have good reason to be worried about all of these life issues, applying more stringent criteria, such as specifying criteria for the exact nature of the worry as apprehensive expectation (APA, 1994), rather than simply considering the nature of the worry as preoccupation with ongoing life stressors, may be relevant to differentiating between the two conditions. As with depression, it is also possible for CFS and generalized anxiety disorder to coexist in some patients. Friedberg and Jason (1998) suggest that the best way of distinguishing between the two disorders is to identify the most prominent symptom in each. For generalized anxiety disorder, the primary feature is excessive, persistent worry. In CFS, it is severe, debilitating fatigue.

## Case Examples*—Pure-Type Conditions

The following are case examples of individuals diagnosed with pure-type conditions (i.e., thorough psychiatric and medical examinations of these patients revealed no evidence of comorbid psychiatric or medical conditions). The first is an example of a person diagnosed with CFS only and no other medical or psychiatric conditions:

---

* Names and characteristics in all case examples have been disguised to protect privacy.

Jane, a 40-year-old woman, was diagnosed with chronic fatigue syndrome (CFS) by her primary care physician. The patient had been entirely healthy until 7 years ago, when she developed a flu-like illness of sudden onset with a low-grade fever, headaches, sore throat, muscle and joint pains, and a constant feeling of profound fatigue. She described the fatigue to her doctor as "a heavy, dead feeling, like [she had been] hit by a truck." Before the illness, the patient was working between 40 and 50 hours per week as an administrative assistant, managing household duties on her own, and serving as the primary evening caretaker for two children (ages 7 and 10). Since the onset of this illness, she has had to quit her job and can no longer keep up with family-related responsibilities. As a result, her husband has had to cut back on his work hours in order to manage the caretaking and household responsibilities. Meanwhile, the patient's symptoms have not improved and appear to be getting worse. Recently, the patient has noticed that she becomes fatigued to the point that she is bedridden for a full day after previously tolerable levels of exercise (such as grocery shopping or coaching her daughter's volleyball games). Even though the patient sleeps between 10 and 12 hours per night, her sleep is broken, and she usually wakes up in the mornings feeling weak and unrested. As a result, she has begun taking frequent naps during the day, without obtaining relief. She has also begun to feel disoriented and confused at times and has noticed an overall worsening of her short-term memory and concentration, requiring her to rely heavily on calendars and reminder lists of things she must do during the day. She now finds that she is unable to remain standing or sitting upright for any prolonged period without a worsening of symptoms. The patient feels sad and irritable during particularly severe symptom flare-ups and has started to doubt that her condition will ever improve. However, her strong religious faith and supportive family are helping her to cope with the day-to-day struggles that the illness presents. She reported that ways in which she copes include maintaining supportive, loving connection with God, family, and friends; accepting the chronic and variable nature of her condition; educating herself about recent research, including experimental and alternative treatments; and corresponding with other CFS patients by e-mail. Past medical, family, and surgical histories were unremarkable. She did not have any allergies to medications. She has been taking Tylenol and multivitamins. Physical examination revealed tender and slightly enlarged lymph nodes. The rest of the examination and laboratory results were normal.

In this first case example, it is apparent that the patient is experiencing severe, progressive CFS symptoms in the absence of psychiatric disorder. She appears to have maintained a strong sense of self-esteem and to have sustained significant feelings of connection with others despite the debilitating effects of CFS on her body and functioning. The second case example describes a man who has been diagnosed with FMS only and no other medical or psychiatric conditions.

John, a 52-year-old corporate executive, was diagnosed with FMS 1 year ago, when he began to experience intense pain in a variety of muscle groups and tenderness to touch in certain areas near his joints and along his back that he could no longer ignore. Throughout his life, John had been an avid athlete and socially active person, enjoying downhill skiing, water polo, racquetball, playing weekly poker with friends, and eating dinner out at least once a month with his wife and business partners. He also used to enjoy receiving massages following athletics. However, as John became more successful at his job, he began to work longer hours and limit his physical activity. While he made it a point to continue his involvement in poker games, he cut back on athletics and dinners in order to conserve energy and save time. Even during the time when John had the time to be more physically active, he had always experienced minor muscle aches and pains, but he had attributed them to "overdoing it" athletically. As the pain became progressively worse with age and decreases in exercise, John began to wonder whether the pain was attributable to not having engaged in as much exercise as he had before. The pain appeared to be interfering with his ability to get to sleep and remain asleep, and he began to experience frequent headaches. Consequently, John began a regular exercise routine, began to eat a more balanced diet, and sought massage therapy. Despite these adjustments, he quickly found that he could not exercise with the same intensity, or for the same duration and frequency, as he had previously. Moreover, he did not enjoy receiving the kind of deep muscle massage therapy that he used to receive and often had to ask the therapist to alter her technique due to severe, distinctive pain upon pressure to several areas of his body. John quickly found that he was more comfortable with mild aerobic exercise (i.e., brisk walking), stretching, and isometric strength-building exercises, and found that this activity was most beneficial in relieving some of his pain if performed approximately three times per week, but not more than that (or else he experienced an increase in fatigue). As a result of his discovery, John made a point to cut down on his work schedule and engage in these pleasant exercises three times per week. Although these exercises alleviated some of the intensity of the pain in some of the muscle groups, John noticed that he continued to experience widespread muscle pain, and that the pain did not appear to dissipate entirely with exercise. At that point, he consulted his primary care physician, who suspected fibromyalgia and referred him to a rheumatologist, who ultimately diagnosed the condition. John continues to cope with his condition by limiting stress in his life, by cutting back on his work hours and utilizing a work assistant, and by taking .5 mg of Klonopin nightly for pain relief and sleep facilitation.

The second patient, John, also appears to evidence no psychiatric abnormalities. Despite FMS symptoms, he appears to have found a way of coping with his illness that works for him and appears to be functioning at an appropriate level given his limitations. The third case example describes a woman experiencing multiple chemical sensitivities and no other medical or psychiatric conditions. During the psychiatric evaluation, a diagnosis of atypical phobia was ruled out, thus confirming a pure-type diagnosis of MCS:

Jacqueline, a 35-year-old woman and former photography instructor at a junior college, was diagnosed with multiple chemical sensitivities (MCS) 5 years ago. Following an accidental spill of a large container of developing fluid in the photography studio at the college where she worked, Jacqueline immediately developed a number of symptoms of MCS including severe nausea; dizziness; a rash on her arms, neck, and chest; and mild difficulty breathing. She left work immediately, and all of her symptoms except the rash dissipated by breakfast time the next morning. However, when Jacqueline returned to the photo lab to work the next day, she began to feel ill instantly and had to leave work even though all of the fluid had been mopped up the previous day. This pattern continued to ebb and flow for the remainder of the week, and Jacqueline began to notice that she was not only feeling ill at work but was also experiencing headaches, nausea, and increased irritability while sitting in city traffic and when cleaning her bathroom and kitchen. She sought treatment from her primary care physician, who referred her to an allergist. Following a series of tests, the allergist suspected MCS and recommended that Jacqueline take a leave of absence from work. Despite this leave of absence, Jacqueline continued to feel ill whenever she encountered road traffic and also noticed that she was sensitive to her own perfumes (when she had not been before). After attempting to return to work several weeks later and continuing to experience the same symptoms as before, Jacqueline had to quit her job permanently and seek vocational counseling to assist her with a career change. In addition, Jacqueline strictly had to limit all contact with certain chemical exposures, including diesel fuels from trucks and buses encountered in city traffic and at the airport, most cleaning products, and perfumes. Given that she graduated from college with a degree in English literature and had sound writing skills, Jacqueline was successful in finding a new job as a book editor. She removed all chemical products that she was sensitive to from her home, she adjusted her schedule such that she no longer traveled during rush-hour traffic, and she was able successfully to avoid other environmental toxins that exacerbated her condition to approximate her premorbid social, emotional, and occupational functioning.

As with the first two patients, Jacqueline clearly depicts an individual who learned how to cope with and adjust to some extremely debilitating and bothersome physical symptoms. It is possible that her preexisting intellectual resources and writing skills facilitated a smooth transition to alternative employment, which reduced her overall levels of psychological distress and helped her to maintain a more hopeful and positive outlook.

## Case Examples—CFS, FMS, MCS, and Comorbid Psychiatric Conditions

The following case examples illustrate cases in which individuals are experiencing both a primary illness of CFS, FMS, or MCS and a coexisting psychiatric disorder.

### CFS

At age 59, Nancy had suffered from CFS for 7 years. Her worst symptoms were physical and mental fatigue, memory and concentration problems, general malaise, and shortness of breath after normal activity. Although these symptoms prevented her from working, she remained active by socializing with friends and visiting her three young grandchildren. The psychodiagnostic evaluation excluded any Axis I disorder but did reveal Axis II compulsive traits. In particular, a clean orderly house was so important to her that any deviation from this exacting standard would cause her to straighten up frenetically and repetitively clean. A stress-symptom record revealed in very concrete terms how her excessive attention to the house was exacerbating both stress reactions and CFS symptoms. In addition, the record identified an overwork-collapse pattern with respect to socializing with her friends and going out in general. She tended to do more than was prudent when her symptoms flared and would then suffer postexertional collapses that could result in compelled bed rest for up to 2 weeks. (A cognitive-behavioral intervention for this patient may be found in Chapter 7.)

### FMS

Alison's symptoms began about 15 years ago and now included pain in the hips, shoulders, back, feet, and hands as well as persistent exertion-related fatigue, multijoint pain, and difficulty remembering names. An FMS-related sleep disturbance reduced her restful sleep to 3 or 4 hours a night. A quick acting tranquilizer, Ambien, helped with the sleep disturbance when it became very severe. Now age 38, she had been diagnosed with FMS 4 years ago after numerous medical evaluations that revealed no definitive diagnosis. Alison also suffered from migraine headaches (which are not uncommon in FMS patients) about once a month which could be triggered by stress, bright lights, or eating chocolate. The severity of the headache prevented her from working for 1 or 2 days. A regimen of 20 mg daily Paxil has reduced the migraine frequency from once a week to her current level.

Alison was a dedicated first-grade schoolteacher who enjoyed the challenge of her work although it exhausted her and exacerbated the bodily pain. The job was also important because it paid for her family's health insurance; however, she was beginning to question if she could physically endure the work much longer. The patient maintained an energy-depleting schedule of teaching, family responsibilities for her two children, volunteer work at her church, and housekeeping. Lately, she was feeling overwhelmed by her symptoms as well as her responsibilities. In addition, she was frustrated and angry about her limitations and others' lack of understanding of them.

The patient wanted to do a thorough examination of her lifestyle in order to see what adjustments could be made to ease her symptoms and their impact on her life. Although she had always viewed herself as competent to handle all challenges and responsibilities, her self-perception of invulnerability was becoming increasingly unrealistic. Yet the patient was hesitant to change any aspect of her life. Based on therapy discussions, healthy changes would have included asking for more physical and emotional support from her husband, requesting a reduction of responsibilities in her teaching position, or engaging in any leisurely pursuit, such as playing the guitar, which she had previously enjoyed. She feared disapproval and rejection by expressing these concerns which would reveal her "weaknesses." In addition, Alison thought she should be happy with the status quo, that is, a good marriage, well-adjusted children, and satisfying work. These clinical issues were examined and resolved to a significant degree in a cognitive-behavioral treatment format (see Chapter 7).

## MCS

Carolyn was married for 20 years and had a 5-year-old daughter. Now 43, she had run her own interior design business which involved frequent exposures to paint thinner and turpentine. Three years ago, while silk screening, she began to develop symptoms of mental disorientation and spaciness, irritability, concentration difficulty, slurred speech, and short-temperedness. These neuropsychiatric symptoms eventually prevented her from working and caused conflict with her husband, who initially did not believe she was really sick. Over several months, she developed chronic respiratory difficulties as well. Her symptoms also seemed to be triggered by indoor exposures to pesticides, formaldehyde, mold, and mothballs. As a result, the family moved from house to house in an attempt to find a chemically nontoxic dwelling where her symptoms might not flare up.

The patient's disability caused her to lose her business, which severely strained the family's finances. Her illness and the losses she suffered induced a secondary generalized anxiety disorder, which also resembled agoraphobia. Once Carolyn and her family located and moved into a relatively MCS-safe home, she noticed that her symptoms began to improve. Feeling significantly better she dreaded the next attack of MCS symptoms. She not only began to worry about having symptom relapses but also began to worry about the possibility of her child developing the illness. As a result, she began to fear leaving her home, spent most of her time dusting and vacuuming her home, and would often visualize herself becoming ill upon setting foot in her car (even before turning on the engine). Because many doctors had dismissed her complaints, she was acutely sensitive to any suggestion of psychotherapy made by her husband because she interpreted it as implying that her problem was simply the result of stress or a psychological disorder. Chapter 7 contains a summary of Carolyn's response to cognitive-behavioral treatment.

The preceding cases illustrate the personal travails suffered by individuals with controversial illnesses. Furthermore, these cases show how lifestyle, behavior, belief systems, and personal stress influence the presented symptomatology and impairments.

# CHAPTER 4

# Psychometric and Behavioral Assessment

Given the difficulties with diagnostic ambiguity and symptom overlap discussed in detail in Chapter 3, accurate assessment of CFS, FMS, and MCS should incorporate the following general guidelines:

1. Questions should be open-ended or dimensional and nonbinary. Questions that merely assess the occurrence or nonoccurrence of a symptom are less accurate than those that assess levels of frequency and severity.
2. Assessment should be longitudinal, with repeated measurement of symptoms over time. Many patients, particularly those with CFS, have symptoms that appear and then disappear for extended periods of time. Assessment of particular symptoms at one point may not reveal the same results as assessment of the same symptoms at another point.

CFS, FMS, and MCS should never be diagnosed using self-report questionnaires alone, but such questionnaires can contribute to the comprehensive assessment of these conditions. Therefore, the choice of appropriate rating scales that measure the construct in question and are relevant to the population being studied is paramount. Although a number of measures of fatigue, psychosocial functioning, and disability exist in the literature, those described herein represent the scales most commonly used with the CFS population, as well as those most likely to be applicable for individuals with FMS and MCS.

# Evaluation of Fatigue and Chronic Fatigue Syndrome

Researchers have identified several types of fatigue states, including pain-related fatigue, hypoglycemic fatigue, mental fatigue, allergy-related fatigue, metabolic fatigue, acidosis, muscle fatigue, and hypothyroid fatigue (Dechene et al., 1994). Since the first fatigue rating scale was published in 1969 (Bartley & Chute, 1969), researchers have attempted to quantify fatigue from a variety of perspectives, including subjective, self-report measures as well as in-vivo behavioral measures of actual activity levels (Friedberg & Jason, 1998). Current self-report measures can be grouped into two categories: fatigue intensity measures and fatigue/function measures (Friedberg & Jason, 1998).

## CFS and Fatigue Questionnaires

### The CFS Screening Questionnaire

The CFS Screening Questionnaire is a valid, reliable, and comprehensive screening device developed to detect cases of fatigue within the general population and to serve as a preliminary screening measure of self-reported CFS symptoms (Jason, Ropacki, et al., 1997). It is a longer and more comprehensive questionnaire than the brief diagnostic measure featured in Appendix A (pp. 97–103). The entire questionnaire consists of two parts. Part 1 assesses sociodemographic characteristics, fatigue severity (Chalder et al., 1993), and interference of fatigue with usual daily activities. Part 2 is administered to individuals reporting 6 or more months of chronic fatigue in Part 1. Part 2 assesses for the presence of the eight minor symptoms of CFS (Fukuda et al., 1994) and also measures characteristics associated with fatigue such as fatigue duration, frequency of fatigue, attributions regarding the cause of fatigue, and fatigue-related functional impairment. Part 2 also contains a series of questions assessing previous diagnosis of any other medical or psychiatric conditions associated with chronic fatigue. A copy of this measure is provided in Appendix B (pp. 105–128).

### Fatigue Scale

The Fatigue Scale (Chalder et al., 1993) is a valid and reliable measure of fatigue intensity designed for use by individuals with CFS and other medical illnesses attending outpatient clinics. This 11-item scale contains responses that are rated on a four-option continuum ranging from 0 = less/better than usual to 3 = much more/much worse than usual. The period of time that respondents reflect about their fatigue is the last month. Scores can be summed to provide a total fatigue severity score ranging from 0 to 33 (with higher scores indicating greater fatigue severity). Principal component analysis performed by the scale's authors supported the notion of a two-factor scale for fatigue (physical and mental fatigue). Physical fatigue refers to items such as "Do you have less strength in your muscles?" and mental fatigue referred to items describing cognitive difficulties such as "Do you have difficulty concentrating?" One limitation of the Chalder et al. (1993) Fatigue Scale in terms of assessing CFS is that the scale was designed specifically to assess only symptoms associated with CFS that relate to fatigue, as opposed to CFS symptoms that are not associated with fatigue. Therefore, it should not be used alone as a screening instrument for CFS. A second limitation is that the scale strictly measures fatigue intensity.

*Fatigue Severity Scale*

The Fatigue Severity Scale (Krupp et al., 1989) is a valid measure of the behavioral consequences of fatigue. It is comprised of nine items that are rated according to a Likert-type rating scale from 1 to 7, where 1 indicates no impairment and 7 indicates severe impairment. The items were initially selected to identify common features of fatigue in both multiple sclerosis (MS) and systemic lupus erythematosus (SLE). In the initial validation study (Krupp et al., 1989), individuals with MS and SLE were compared with normal, healthy adults. Internal consistency for the Fatigue Severity Scale was high for both illness groups. Studies of individuals with CFS revealed that Fatigue Severity Scale scores were significantly higher for individuals with CFS, as compared with individuals with MS or primary depression (Pepper et al., 1993). One limitation of the scale is that a ceiling effect may limit its ability to assess severe fatigue-related disability, and the true association between this scale and other health-related measures may be underestimated for this reason (Friedberg & Jason, 1998).

One investigation (Taylor, Jason, & Torres, 2000) explored relationships between these two commonly used fatigue rating scales in CFS research, the Fatigue Scale (Chalder et al., 1993) and the Fatigue Severity Scale (Krupp et al., 1989). Theoretically, these scales have been described as measuring different aspects of the fatigue construct; the Fatigue Scale (Chalder et al., 1993) was developed as a measure of the severity of specific fatigue-related symptoms, while the Fatigue

Severity Scale (Krupp et al., 1989) was designed to assess functional outcomes related to fatigue. Associations of these scales with eight symptoms typically observed in individuals with CFS (Fukuda et al., 1994), and with eight domains of functional disability (Ware & Sherbourne, 1992) were measured among individuals with self-reported, CFS-like symptoms. Findings revealed that the Fatigue Severity Scale (Krupp et al., 1989) appears to represent a more accurate and comprehensive measure of fatigue-related severity, symptomatology, and functional disability for individuals with CFS-like symptomatology.

## Evaluation of Disability and Quality of Life

### Medical Outcomes Study Short Form-36 Health Survey

The Medical Outcomes Study Short Form-36 Health Survey (MOS SF-36) (Ware & Sherbourne, 1992) is a reliable and valid measure that discriminates between gradations of functional impairment. It identifies disability along several dimensions including physical activities, bodily pain, energy and fatigue, perceptions of general health, social functioning, and mental health. The energy and fatigue scale has been used on its own as a rating scale of fatigue intensity for individuals with hypertension, prostate disease, and AIDS, but its brevity may lead to floor effects in severely disabling illnesses such as CFS (Friedberg & Jason, 1998). Perhaps as a result, the energy and fatigue scale has not been widely used in isolation from the other MOS SF-36 scales in CFS research.

Depending on the scale, items are scored in Likert-type format, with scores ranging from 1-2, 1-3, 1-5, or 1-6. Item raw scores are then converted to scaled scores, and scaled scores are then summed to form an overall score for each scale, as described in the scoring manual (Medical Outcomes Trust, 1994). Overall, higher scores indicate better health or less functional impairment. Reliability and validity studies of the MOS SF-36 have shown adequate internal consistency, discriminant validity among subscales, and substantial differences between patient and nonpatient populations in the pattern of scores (McHorney et al., 1994; McHorney, Ware, & Raczek, 1993). It has demonstrated adequate psychometric properties as a measure of functional status in a population of individuals with CFS, and it has distinguished CFS from other fatiguing illnesses (Buchwald et al., 1996).

## Quality of Life Index

The Quality of Life Index (Ferrans & Powers, 1985, 1992) is a 72-item scale that is used effectively to measure perceived overall quality of life among individuals with CFS (Anderson & Ferrans, 1997). The Quality of Life Index measures quality of life in four major domains: health and functioning, social and economic, psychological/spiritual, and family. This instrument differs from most other measures in its acknowledgment that individuals place different priority on different aspects of life quality. What one person considers a disability may merely represent a nuisance for another (Ferrans, 1990). The Quality of Life Index was designed to account for the observation that people differ with respect to which aspects of life quality they value the most such that life quality dimensions do not impact equally on perceptions of overall quality of life. The Quality of Life Index is comprised of two corresponding sections. One measures a person's satisfaction with 34 aspects of life on a 6-point Likert-type scale (ranging from "very dissatisfied" to "very satisfied"), and the other measures the importance of those same aspects to the individual on a similar 6-point Likert-type scale (ranging from "very unimportant" to "very important").

# Evaluating Psychosocial Phases of Illness and Coping

## The Fennell Phase Inventory

The Fennell Phase Inventory is a 20-item questionnaire designed to assess four psychosocial phases of the illness experience (Jason, Fennell, et al., 1999). Five items are used to measure each of the four phases. Each item is rated on a 5-point scale (1 = definitely do not agree, 5 = very strongly agree). Recent studies suggest that this inventory appears to be a promising way of differentiating the phases that are experienced by patients with CFS (Jason, Fennell, et al., 1999). Although it has only undergone formal evaluation using individuals with CFS, Patricia Fennell has suggested that the four phases model can be applied to individuals with other chronic illnesses, including FMS and MCS. The four phases measured by this inventory include Crisis, Stabilization, Resolution, and Integration (Fennell, 1993). In Phase 1, the "Crisis Phase," patients physically move from the initial onset of CFS to an eventual crisis state, wherein they respond with uncertainty and emotional distress to the trauma of a new illness. In Phase 2, the "Stabilization Phase," patients continue to experience physical and behavioral chaos and dissembling, followed by an eventual stabilization characterized by some recognition and predictability of their symptoms. In Phase 3, the "Resolution Phase," patients work to accept the chronicity and ambiguity of their illness and create meaning out of the illness experience. Phase 3 is characterized by plateau, relapse, or progression, all constituting the normal cycling of chronic illness. In the final stage, the "Integration Phase," patients advance to a state of integration, where they are able to integrate pre- and postillness self-concepts and sometimes psychologically transcend the CFS illness. They realize they may either continue to cycle, or their health may improve significantly. Patients often construct a new identity: a combination of themselves before and after the illness experience. A copy of the Fennell Phase Inventory and scoring procedures is provided in Appendix D (pp. 131–134).

## Fatigue-Related Cognitions Scale

The Fatigue-Related Cognitions Scale (Friedberg & Krupp, 1994) contained in Appendix C (pp. 129–130), is a 14-item scale specifically developed to measure dysfunctional beliefs about the symptom of fatigue among individuals with CFS, and it is able to distinguish between individuals with CFS and those with primary depression (with individuals with CFS scoring higher). The scale contains a 5-point response format that asks patients about their cognitive reactions to fatigue symptoms. Stress-related maladaptive thinking can be identified with this measure. Examples of items include "I think about my fatigue often," "My fatigue makes me angry," and "I sometimes think I deserve the fatigue I feel." It has been evaluated as an excellent tool for rapid clinical assessment of beliefs about fatigue in individuals with CFS (Friedberg & Jason, 1998).

## The Illness Management Questionnaire

The Illness Management Questionnaire (IMQ) (Ray et al., 1993) was developed specifically to assess coping in individuals with CFS and has been used extensively in studies of adults with CFS (Ray, Jefferies, & Weir, 1995). The IMQ has four factors: Maintaining Activity (attempting to ignore symptoms, disregarding possible adverse effects of activity), Accommodating to the Illness (organizing and arranging one's life to avoid exertion and manage stress), Focusing on Symptoms (preoccupation with symptoms, viewing one's life as dominated by the illness), and Information Seeking (searching for relevant information and an openness to try treatments). Higher scores indicate more agreement with the items measured in each domain. It is possible that this instrument could be used to assess coping in individuals with FMS and MCS as well.

## Evaluating Stigmatizing Attitudes

### Chronic Fatigue Syndrome Attitudes Test

The Chronic Fatigue Syndrome Attitudes Test (CAT) (Shlaes, Jason, & Ferrari, 1999) is a valid and reliable measure designed to assess knowledge and attributions regarding CFS among individuals who do not have CFS. This 19-item scale was created using several constructs outlined in the literature regarding negative attitudes toward people with CFS, disabilities, and AIDS. The first factor, "Responsibility for CFS," contains items relating to whether respondents feel that people with CFS are responsible for getting sick. The second factor, "Relevance of CFS," contains items relating to the public importance of CFS. The third factor, "Traits of People With CFS," contains items relating to perceptions about personality characteristics of individuals with CFS. Eight other items were used as distracter items but were not used to score the CAT. The CAT subscales and composite scale have demonstrated excellent internal consistency, and test-retest reliability analysis demonstrated that the CAT subscale scores, as well as the CAT composite score, were consistent over a 6-week period. A copy of the CAT and scoring procedures is presented in Appendix E (pp. 135–137).

## Assessing Psychiatric Comorbidity in CFS, FMS, and MCS

Because many CFS symptoms match the criteria for certain psychiatric disorders (e.g., depression, anxiety, and somatoform disorders), a careful psychiatric assessment that accurately weighs the contribution of physiologic and psychiatric factors is essential in guiding the diagnosis and eventual treatment of CFS patients. Few current approaches to psychiatric assessment used in research studies effectively meet the challenge of achieving a true diagnostic picture and incorporating the complexities of a patient's illness experience. Symptom rating scales, such as the Beck Depression Inventory (BDI; Beck, 1967), and standardized diagnostic interviews, such as the Diagnostic Interview Schedule (DIS; Robins et al., 1989), most commonly used in CFS research, tend to overdiagnose psychiatric illness in CFS patients (Taylor & Jason, 1998).

### Structured Clinical Interview for the *DSM-IV*

The Structured Clinical Interview for the *DSM-IV* (SCID; First et al., 1995) is a professionally administered, semistructured psychiatric interview that will be used to diagnose Axis I psychiatric disorders according to *DSM-IV* criteria. In contrast to other measures of psychiatric disorders that do not allow for the incorporation of context-specific information, the SCID allows for clinical judgment in the assignment of symptoms to psychiatric or medical categories, a crucial distinction in the assessment of symptoms that overlap between CFS and psychiatric disorders (Friedberg & Jason, 1998). Symptoms within each diagnostic category are scored as either absent, subthreshold, or present, and all symptoms that are present are counted toward the diagnostic tally as it conforms to *DSM-IV* criteria.

### Evaluation of FMS and MCS

Albert Donnay (1998) has developed a scale designed to screen for, but not to diagnose, FMS and MCS. Although the scale does not assess for the exact research criteria for FMS put forth by Wolfe and associates (1990), it offers a good starting point for the detection of FMS-related symptomatology. In addition, White et al. (1999) developed an empirically valid screening instrument designed to identify potential cases of FMS within a London general population. This scale was found to demonstrate adequate sensitivity and specificity and was determined to be useful in screening for FMS in nonclinical populations. Donnay's (1998) questionnaire items assessing FMS and MCS are contained in the CFS Screening Questionnaire in Appendix B (pp. 105–128).

## Evaluating Service Utilization in CFS, FMS, and MCS

Utilization of appropriate services can represent an important aspect of any treatment regimen for individuals with CFS, FMS, and MCS. The Service Utilization Checklist, employed in a needs assessment study of individuals with CFS (Jason et al., 1996), is a measure of the frequency of utilization of services and resources most commonly used by individuals with fatigue-related disorders. This checklist takes between 2 to 5 minutes to complete, and it is scored by summing the frequencies of each service utilized for a total service utilization score. Higher scores indicate greater service utilization.

## Physical Activity Monitoring in CFS and FMS

Monitoring of physical activity can be an essential component of any treatment plan regimen (refer to Chapter 7). Two common forms of in-vivo behavioral activity monitoring include actigraphy and pedometer use. An actigraph is a device worn on the belt that provides numeric data quantifying multidimensional aspects of movement. A pedometer is a less sophisticated and less expensive device also worn on the belt that provides an assessment of the number of steps an individual takes. Pedometers can be used as an assessment tool for interventions in clinical settings (refer to Chapter 6).

# CHAPTER 5

# Pharmacological and Alternative Treatments

Pharmacological and alternative treatments represent two avenues that may lead to alleviation of the severity of some, but not all, of the symptoms of CFS, FMS, and MCS. Most of the treatments covered in this section have not been adequately studied (Reid et al., 2000), and preliminary studies have demonstrated varying degrees of efficacy depending upon the patient group and the specific symptom being treated. It should be cautioned that none of the treatments discussed in this section was developed specifically to treat these controversial illnesses and are likely to be palliative at best in treating particular symptoms (e.g., pain, sleep, headache, and possibly fatigue and cognitive problems in some circumstances), rather than the entire illness, per se. Ongoing consultation with and careful monitoring by a physician or alternative medicine specialist highly experienced in the treatment of these conditions are strongly recommended for any patient who is interested in these treatments.

Regardless of the medication described, it is important to note that very few pharmacological agents have been well established as effective for these conditions (Reid et al., 2000), and what works well for one person may not be tolerated by, or may be ineffective for another person. Reports by patients of hypersensitivity reactions to even small doses of the medications described on the following pages (particularly antidepressants) are not unusual among individuals with these conditions (Friedberg, 1996; Verrillo & Gellman, 1997). Some suggest that physicians who prescribe medications for patients with CFS, FMS, and MCS should start at lower than normal dosages and increase slowly only if they are well tolerated (Donnay, 1998).

- *Prozac.* Prozac (fluoxetine) is an antidepressant medication that has been used to treat these controversial illnesses through its direct influence on levels and action of the neurotransmitter, serotonin. For individuals with these conditions, Prozac is thought to increase the availability of serotonin, hence reducing excessive sleep, severe depression, and pain. Prozac appears to have variable effectiveness on individuals with CFS, FMS, and MCS, with some researchers finding evidence for significant improvement in symptoms and functioning, and others finding no benefit on fatigue or any other somatic symptoms. A recent review of treatment research found few randomized controlled trials and insufficient evidence to support the use of antidepressants to directly treat many of the symptoms of CFS. Two randomized clinical trials of Prozac did not show efficacy for symptoms of CFS or depression (Reid et al., 2000). A review of FMS treatment studies indicated that antidepressants, including Prozac, did not result in meaningful improvements in psychological status and daily functioning in the few studies that included these as outcome variables (Rossy et al., 1999). Moreover, these researchers found that nonpharmacological forms of treatment (i.e., cognitive behavior therapy) were superior to pharmacological treatment with respect to self-report of FMS symptoms and functioning. While some individuals with CFS, FMS, and MCS have reported some positive effects resulting from Prozac, others (at least 15%) have been completely unable to tolerate its side effects, which may include worsening of insomnia and disruption in stage-four delta sleep, paradoxical excessive sedation, anxiety, agitation, and severe gastrointestinal problems. According to Starlanyl and Copeland (1996), symptoms of FMS sometimes worsen with Prozac due to the disruption of stage-four sleep.
- *Klonopin.* Klonopin (clonazepam) is a benzodiazepine and antiseizure agent that acts directly on the limbic system, thalamus, and hypothalamus to reduce anxiety, facilitate sleep, improve cognitive functioning, and control muscle twitching (myoclonus), muscle pain, restless legs syndrome, and nighttime grinding of teeth in individuals with CFS and FMS. Clinical anecdotes suggest that Klonopin is effective in treating a number of CFS and FMS symptoms, and has relatively mild

side effects (sedation, excessive thirst, depression, and gastrointestinal upset for some individuals). However, Klonopin has not undergone systematic study in these controversial illnesses.

- *Serzone.* As part of a sleep-wake intervention for individuals with CFS proposed by Hickie and Davenport (1999) Serzone (nefazodone) is a serotonin-2 receptor antagonist administered at night to assist with sleep onset and quality. Serzone is an antidepressant that is structurally different from other antidepressants because it increases levels of two neurotransmitters, serotonin and norepinephrine. Although this agent has antidepressant properties, antidepressant effects are not the major reason for its utility with individuals with CFS and its potential utility for individuals with FMS. It should be noted that Serzone has not undergone systematic study in randomized controlled trials with individuals with CFS, FMS, or MCS.

- *Ampligen.* Ampligen is an experimental medication that has demonstrated some efficacy in the treatment of certain symptoms in certain types of individuals with CFS (Suhadolnik, Reichenbach, Hitzges, Adelson, et al., 1994; Suhadolnik, Reichenbach, Hitzges, Sobol, et al., 1994). However, it is a highly controversial drug that has also been anecdotally reported to be associated with highly negative long-term physical health consequences (Kansky, 2000). By definition, Ampligen is a mismatched double-stranded ribonucleic acid that can serve as an immune system modulator and antiviral agent for some individuals with CFS. Ampligen is thought to treat the low latent 2-5A synthetase and upregulated RNase (ribonuclease) L activity found in some individuals with CFS (Suhadolnick, Reichenbach, Hitzges, Adelson, et al., 1994; Suhadolnick, Reichenbach, Hitzges, Sobol, et al., 1994). While still evolving, current treatment requires two intravenous infusions per week over a 9- to 16-month period (Verrillo & Gellman, 1997), with longer treatment periods appearing to produce more long-term benefits. Potential benefits reported by patients with sudden illness onset, significant limitations in performing activities of daily living, and cognitive impairment include significant increases in energy and the ability to perform activities of daily living, reduction in pain, return of immune system functioning to normal range, and significant improvement in cognitive functioning.

It is important to note that this drug is still in an experimental phase, and the exact percentage of patients who will benefit substantially, if at all in the long term, is yet to be determined. In short-term studies, use of Ampligen has been found to produce the following side effects, which tend to occur during the first 3 months of treatment: initial worsening of nausea, dizziness, headaches, and pain. Ampligen is available within the United States and Brussels on an experimental basis only. It is extremely cost-prohibitive. One year of treatment currently costs over $14,500. Thus, not all individuals with CFS will have access to this medication. More information about Ampligen can be found at the following website: http://www.cfs-news.org/ampligen.htm.

## Alternative Medical Approaches

### Body Work

Acupuncture is a Chinese therapeutic technique that involves the insertion of small, solid needles under the skin at vital life energy points (called "chi" points) at different depths in order to raise endorphin levels and thereby promote major organ repair, correct chemical imbalances, regulate body metabolism, and restore the body's harmony. According to the Chinese theoretical orientation, vital life energy flows throughout the body and can be felt along specific meridians, or imaginary lines along which the needles are ultimately inserted. When a person becomes ill, these paths or meridians become tender or painful. Insertion of needles at these points is thought to signal the brain to send healing energy to that area. According to Verrillo and Gellman (1997), about half of the patients with CFS they surveyed tried acupuncture, and half of that group reported the following improvements: reduced general pain, reduced eye pain, improvement in overall well-being, and increased mental clarity and energy. Approximately one-third reported negative results, including overstimulated immune system, severe relapse, and intolerance, and a smaller proportion reported no results.

Verrillo and Gellman (1997) contend that positive results of acupuncture are often achieved when treatment aims to correct very specific problems, such as pain, insomnia, loss of appetite, or nausea. However, negative results may be attributable to a mistaken belief by the acupuncturist that individuals with CFS have depressed immune functioning (when the opposite, overactive immune functioning, has been supported by research and is more likely the correct hypothesis). Assuming underactive immune functioning, the acupuncturist may cause excess stimulation to the immune symptoms, thereby causing profound symptom exacerbation. Acupuncture is seldom used alone in Asia but instead is typically used in combination with Shiatsu massage and herbal remedies. Acupuncture is the treatment of choice for FMS in Brazil (Starlanyl & Copeland, 1996) and may also be of particular value to individuals with MCS and numerous allergies (Verrillo & Gellman, 1997). One cautionary note is that acupuncture is not innocuous. An inexperienced or misinformed acupuncturist can trigger a relapse. One means of determining the expertise of one's practitioner is to check with the National Commission for the Certification of Acupuncturists to ensure certification. Other important areas to assess include whether the acupuncturist uses new needles with each treatment; duration of experience practicing acupuncture; past experience treating individuals with CFS, FMS, or MCS; and references from other individuals with CFS, FMS, or MCS that the acupuncturist has treated.

Acupressure (G-Jo) is another Chinese therapy used in the immediate treatment of minor illnesses. It relies on noninvasive stimulation of certain points on the skin using light pressure by the fingertips to release vital life energy (chi). Acupressure can potentially be used in the treatment of mild to moderate symptoms of CFS, including muscle pain, insomnia, shortness of breath, nausea, headache, eyestrain, and associated tension and anxiety (Verrillo & Gellman, 1997). Because it has not been formally evaluated in treatment studies, consultation with the patient's physician should precede any recommendation for this type of treatment (Verrillo & Gellman, 1997).

## Massage

Research in the field of massage therapy has provided empirical support for the efficacy of massage in treating many of the symptoms of chronic fatigue syndrome and fibromyalgia, including reducing pain and fatigue, increasing mental alertness, and enhancing immune function (Field, 1998).

**Nutritional Supports**

No systematic evaluation of nutritional supports in CFS has occurred (Reid et al., 2000). Based largely on anecdotal and clinical evidence, Verrillo and Gellman (1997) suggest that certain nutritional supports or supplements may serve to relieve some symptoms for certain types of patients with CFS, FMS, and MCS. Commonly used agents include SAM-e, malic acid, magnesium, and NADH (the reduced form of nicotinamide adenine dinucleotide). Patients should always consult a physician before introducing any of these substances into their treatment regimens.

SAM-e (S-adenosylmethionine), a synthetic replication of a natural metabolite of the amino acid methionine, is an antiinflammatory drug with analgesic and antidepressant effects. On a cellular level, SAM-e maintains mitochondrial function, prevents DNA mutations, and restores cellular membrane fluidity so that cell receptors are better able to bind hormones and other factors. Six clinical studies, including two controlled trials, of SAM-e in FMS have shown significant improvements in physical status, self-reported FMS symptoms, and psychological status (Rossy et al., 1999). Clinical anecdote also indicates that SAM-e may be associated with reduced joint and muscle pain and improvements in mood among patients with CFS.

NADH is an important coenzyme in the body because it plays an essential role in the energy production of cells. Research indicates that NADH not only acts as a driving force in the production of cellular energy but also acts as a potent antioxidant, plays a central part in DNA repair and cellular regeneration, and stimulates the production of neurotransmitters, including dopamine, serotonin, and noradrenaline. Current models for neurodegenerative diseases that involve oxidative stress use toxins specific for particular regions of the brain. These toxins are thought to lead to DNA damage and to cell death. Although it has not been well studied, NADH may be of benefit in the treatment of CFS. NADH has been hypothesized to help correct the metabolic defect in CFS that inhibits the production of ATP (adenosine triphosphate) and deprives individuals with CFS of needed energy. NADH may not only reduce fatigue in CFS, but the three neurotransmitters stimulated by NADH production may serve to improve cognitive functioning by improving short-term memory, increasing alertness, reducing negative mood, and improving sleep. Results of early research of the effects of NADH on CFS symptoms have indicated that some individuals with CFS can experience relief from fatigue, increased strength and endurance, and improved mental and physical functioning, with no adverse reactions noted (Forsyth et al., 1999). Results of a larger, FDA-approved clinical trial of the effectiveness of NADH in CFS treatment conducted by the same research group at the Georgetown Medical Center (Dr. Harry Preuss and Dr. Joseph Bellanti) are pending.

Malic acid is a dietary supplement found in apples, pears, and other fruits that serves as an intermediate of the energy-producing Krebs cycle and aids in the production of ATP. It is especially effective in decreasing aluminum toxicity in the brain, as common in Alzheimer's disease, and treatment with malic acid has been shown to reduce the concentration of aluminum found in various organs and tissues. For individuals with CFS and FMS, it is hypothesized to relieve many of the symptoms associated with tissue acidosis, such as muscle spasms, cramps, and burning pain. Some physicians who treat CFS recommend malic acid in combination with magnesium supplements (Verrillo & Gellman, 1997). It is relatively risk free, with the only reported side effect being diarrhea attributable to increased magnesium. Super malic, a combination of malic acid and magnesium, has been used as a treatment for FMS in two clinical studies with mixed results (Rossy et al., 1999).

Research has shown that individuals with CFS and FMS may be deficient in certain compounds required for the synthesis of ATP. One of the most critical elements for ATP production is magnesium, and low levels of magnesium can result in anorexia, PMS, headaches, muscle cramping, nausea, learning disabilities, personality changes, weakness, exhaustion, muscle spasms, heart palpitations, and even heart attacks. Magnesium is a major mineral essential to bodily function in humans. It serves to relay nervous system impulses and facilitate normal metabolism of calcium and potassium, and functions as a coenzyme. Magnesium has also been linked to improvements in heart functioning and sleep. Clinical anecdote supports use of magnesium in the treatment of pain relief, muscle weakness, and fatigue in CFS and FMS. One randomized double-blind placebo controlled study of intramuscular magnesium sulfate injections in 32 individuals with CFS documented significant improvements in energy, diminished pain, and reduced emotional reactions, but these findings have not been replicated (Reid et al., 2000). It should be noted that neither malic acid nor magnesium has undergone systematic evaluation in the treatment of CFS or MCS. According to Reid and associates (2000), limited data from small, randomized controlled trials provide no sustained, replicable evidence of benefit to individuals with CFS from magnesium injections. Finally, oral supplementation with carnitine, an essential fatty acid, has been associated with significant symptomatic improvements in two controlled studies of patients with CFS although a recent randomized clinical trial of essential fatty acids failed to replicate these earlier findings. As with all therapies described in this book, a physician should be consulted to determine proper administration and dosage.

## Patient Ratings of Treatment Efficacy

One study (Friedberg et al., 1994) of individuals with CFS assessed patient ratings of the efficacy of various therapeutic interventions tried. Findings are reprinted with permission in Table 2 on page 59 (Friedberg, 1995), which shows CFS patient rankings of treatment effectiveness for 29 listed medical and alternative therapies. Ampligen was rated as leading to moderate to major improvement in 100% of the three individuals who reported undergoing treatment, and two other interventions, antiallergy diet and antiyeast diet, were more highly rated than were the vast majority of pharmacologic therapies.

A second study (LeRoy, Haney Davis, & Jason, 1996) surveyed 305 individuals with MCS, 41% of whom also had CFS. Table 3 (pp. 60–62) presents ratings of the most and least effective treatments utilized for MCS. In treatments specifically designed for people with MCS, 93% reported benefit from chemical sensitivity avoidance, and 86% were helped by creating environmentally safe homes. Parenthetical numbers in Table 3 represent question numbers on the original survey used in the LeRoy et al. (1996) study.

## Table 2: Treatment Effectiveness Rated by Individuals With CFS*

| Sample Size** | Treatment Tried | Moderate-Major Improvement (%) | Felt Worse (%) |
|---|---|---|---|
| 3 | Ampligen | 100 | 0 |
| 186 | Antiallergy diet | 32 | < 1 |
| 249 | Antidepressent medications | 28 | 31 |
| 183 | Antiyeast diet | 27 | 5 |
| 133 | Stress reduction/biofeedback | 26 | < 1 |
| 114 | IV vitamins/injections | 26 | 4 |
| 180 | Physical therapy/massage | 26 | 16 |
| 109 | Acupuncture | 25 | 10 |
| 60 | Kutapressin | 25 | 12 |
| 65 | Macrobiotic diet | 23 | 15 |
| 184 | Psychotherapy | 19 | 7 |
| 283 | Vitamin/mineral/amino acid therapy | 18 | 5 |
| 127 | Allergy shots | 17 | 27 |
| 129 | Homeopathy | 16 | 12 |
| 112 | Tagamet or other H2 blocker | 16 | 13 |
| 80 | Malic acid | 16 | 14 |
| 76 | Gamma globulin | 16 | 20 |
| 38 | IV antibiotics | 16 | 39 |
| 207 | Anti-inflammatory drugs | 14 | 16 |
| 81 | Antiviral drugs | 14 | 19 |
| 195 | Oral antibiotics | 14 | 36 |
| 55 | Removal of amalgam fillings | 13 | 9 |
| 55 | Magnesium injections | 13 | 11 |
| 184 | Herbal remedies | 13 | 15 |
| 161 | CoEnzyme Q10 | 11 | 13 |
| 10 | Transfer factor | 10 | 30 |
| 44 | Nitroglycerin | 9 | 25 |
| 26 | Alpha/Beta Interferon | 8 | 23 |
| 17 | Chelation therapy | 6 | 12 |

---

\* **Note.** From *Coping With Chronic Fatigue Syndrome: Nine Things You Can Do* (pp. 23-24), by F. Friedberg, 1995, Oakland, CA: New Harbinger. Copyright © 1995 by New Harbinger. Reprinted with permission.

\*\* Sample sizes equal to or greater than 25 yield more reliable results.

## Table 3: Patient Ratings of Treatment Efficacy for MCS*

| Treatment by Category | N | % Helped |
|---|---|---|
| *Treatments Specifically for MCS* | | |
| Chemical sensitivity avoidance (2) | 304 | 93 |
| Create environmentally safe home, if able (3) | 239 | 86 |
| Move to a less polluted area (4) | 145 | 76 |
| Food allergy diet (1) | 299 | 75 |
| Air filters (8) | 270 | 50 |
| Health Med-like sauna detox (7) | 83 | 39 |
| Neutralizations to chemicals (6) | 189 | 22 |
| Neutralizations to foods (5) | 186 | 19 |
| | | |
| *Education, Support, and Growth* | | |
| Reading information about MCS (9) | 303 | 81 |
| Meeting other MCS people (11) | 281 | 69 |
| Joining a support group (10) | 200 | 56 |
| Therapy/Counseling (12)· | 172 | 37 |
| | | |
| *General Supportive Therapies* | | |
| Meditation/Relaxation/Prayer (18) | 267 | 55 |
| Vitamin/Mineral supplements (16) | 290 | 48 |
| Herbal supplements (17) | 217 | 39 |
| Homeopathy (13) | 187 | 36 |
| Chiropractic manipulation (15) | 181 | 33 |
| Acupuncture (14) | 132 | 26 |
| | | |
| *Specific Therapies* | | |
| Antifungal candida therapy (19) | 234 | 41 |
| Avoid electromagnetic fields (21) | 165 | 33 |
| Mercury amalgam removal (20) | 112 | 28 |
| Parasite therapy (22) | 82 | 28 |
| Coffee enemas (24) | 47 | 28 |
| Colonics (23) | 70 | 24 |
| Juicing (35) | 75 | 23 |
| Ultra-Clear (41) | 66 | 18 |
| Hydrogen peroxide therapy (43) | 59 | 12 |

*Data derived from "Treatment Efficacy: A Survey of 305 MCS Patients," by J. Leroy, T. Haney Davis, and L. A. Jason, 1996, *The CFIDS Chronicle, Winter,* pp. 52-53. Copyright © 1996 by The CFIDS Association of America, Inc. Reprinted with permission.

| Treatment by Category | N | % Helped |
|---|---|---|
| *Supplements* | | |
| Vitamin C: Non-ester (29) | 221 | 43 |
| Digestive enzymes (34) | 212 | 35 |
| Vitamin C: Ester (28) | 161 | 34 |
| DHEA (38) | 57 | 30 |
| Thyroid supplements (37) | 147 | 30 |
| Acidophilus (33) | 248 | 30 |
| Echinacea (36) | 163 | 26 |
| Garlic (Kyolic) (31) | 168 | 25 |
| Coenzyme Q10 (normal dose) (32) | 137 | 21 |
| L-Glutathione (reduced) (39) | 80 | 20 |
| Garlic (raw) (30) | 158 | 17 |
| Sunrider herbal products (40) | 46 | 7 |
| KM (42) | 35 | 6 |
| *Antifungal Drugs* | | |
| Diflucan (27) | 77 | 32 |
| Nystatin (25) | 189 | 22 |
| Nizerol (26) | 67 | 19 |
| *Immune System/Antiviral Therapies* | | |
| Vitamin C IV therapy (44) | 110 | 34 |
| Enzyme potentiated desens-EPD (47) | 21 | 33 |
| Transfer factor (50) | 21 | 33 |
| Gamma globulin IV therapy (49) | 11 | 27 |
| Acyclovir (Zovirax) (45) | 32 | 19 |
| Gamma globulin shots (48) | 41 | 18 |
| Kutapressin shots (46) | 9 | 11 |
| *Prescription Drugs* | | |
| Prozac (51) | 50 | 18 |
| Wellbutrin (54) | 12 | 17 |
| Zoloft (52) | 32 | 16 |
| Klonopin (56) | 17 | 12 |
| Sinequan (55) | 32 | 9 |
| Elavil (53) | 62 | 8 |

| Treatment by Category | N | % Helped |
|---|---|---|
| *Chronic Fatigue Syndrome Treatments* | | |
| Stress reduction (58) | 208 | 63 |
| Rest (57) | 229 | 60 |
| Magnesium shots (59) | 57 | 35 |
| High-dose B12 shots (60) | 89 | 35 |
| High-dose coq10 sublingual (61) | 21 | 24 |
| Jesse Stoff approach to CFS (62) | 6 | 0 |

# CHAPTER 6
# Cognitive-Behavioral Treatment I

Activity pacing, or "envelope theory" (Jason, Melrose, et al., 1999), can serve as an effective form of behavioral intervention in the treatment of individuals with CFS and FMS. Unlike other forms of cognitive behavior therapy applied to the treatment of CFS (Sharpe et al., 1996), therapy using envelope theory does not challenge patients' beliefs in a medical cause for their illness. Instead, envelope theory recommends that patients pace their activity according to their available energy resources. In this approach, the phrase "staying within the envelope" is used to designate a comfortable range of energy expenditure in which an individual avoids both overexertion and underexertion, maintaining a more consistent level of activity over time. If a comfortable level of activity is maintained over time, the functional and health status of individuals will slowly improve, and they will find themselves able to engage in increasing levels of activity.

Jason, Melrose, and associates (1999), King and associates (1997), and Pesek, Jason, and Taylor (2000) presented data on the use of this theory during interventions involving repeated self-ratings of perceived and expended energy over time. Findings indicated that when the participants' perceived and expended energy levels were maintained within close proximity (within the envelope), the participants experienced decreases in fatigue over time. Using principles of psychoneuroimmunology, treatment with the envelope theory provides a transactional model, supporting complex interactions between multiple biological and psychological factors that influence the onset of CFS and pathways to further illness or recovery.

Therapy based on envelope theory can be combined with cognitive coping skills therapy (Friedberg, 1995) to treat individuals within a wide range of functioning. As covered in Chapter 7 of this volume, cognitive coping skills therapy focuses on the identification of symptom relapse triggers and encourages activity moderation to minimize setbacks. This therapy also emphasizes cognitive and behavioral coping skills, stress reduction techniques, and social support in an attempt to promote self-regulation and management of CFS symptoms. Unlike some forms of cognitive-behavioral therapy (Sharpe et al., 1996), cognitive coping skills therapy does not challenge or question patients' beliefs in a medical cause for CFS, and it is sensitive to individual differences in activity tolerance. Practitioners using envelope theory and cognitive coping skills therapy are encouraged to respond to patients' symptom accounts with complete empathy and validation for the illness. The following is a case example of therapy which integrates concepts of envelope theory and cognitive coping skills in the treatment of a patient with CFS.

## Case Study Illustrating the Integration of Envelope Theory With Cognitive Behavior Therapy

Carmen is a 38-year-old, divorced woman of third-generation Mexican-American origin who lives alone in a low-income, inner city, Latino neighborhood. Carmen had been working as a bilingual legal assistant until 4 years ago, when she had to leave her job and collect disability income because episodes of debilitating fatigue and chronic pain rendered her unable to complete an adequate amount of work for her employer. Carmen currently remains unemployed and receives social security disability income for her diagnosed condition, chronic fatigue syndrome. With the exception of severe seasonal hay fever and a food allergy to monosodium glutamate, she was a relatively healthy person before she became ill. She has no history of prior mental health treatment.

Carmen became ill with chronic fatigue syndrome 4 years ago following an episode of infectious mononucleosis. After resting for approximately 4 weeks, she began to feel better, and had regained about 60% to 70% of her premono energy. Although not fully recovered, she then returned to work and noticed that she was experiencing difficulty in a number of work performance areas. She attributed these difficulties to low energy levels and a number of cognitive problems, including short-term memory loss, problems concentrating, and difficulties with verbal expression both in English and in Spanish (e.g., slips of the tongue, word-finding difficulties). Over the next 6 months, debilitating levels of fatigue persisted, and she developed severe pain in multiple joints and muscles throughout her body; muscle weakness; exercise intolerance; unrefreshing sleep; and constant, unusual headaches.

During the first 7 months of the illness, Carmen visited three outpatient medical clinics where three different physicians saw her. None of the doctors was able to provide her with a definitive diagnosis or adequate treatment for her condition. Results of physical examination and routine laboratory tests were consistently normal. One physician suggested that her fatigue was related to stress and recommended psychotherapy, one suggested it was due to muscle deconditioning resulting from her sedentary office job and recommended exercise, and the third physician recommended various trials of psychotropic medications, which she tried, with no relief. Only one of the physicians spent longer than 30 minutes examining her, and none of them thought she had "anything serious to worry about." Carmen came away from these doctor visits feeling invalidated, misunderstood, and stigmatized. She began to wonder if her gender and ethnic identity were, in some way, influencing the doctors' behavior and suggestions that the illness was of psychiatric nature.

As time progressed, Carmen's condition worsened. She began to suffer mild fevers, other noticeable and sudden changes in body temperature, chronic sore throats, and painful lymph nodes on an almost daily basis. These symptoms forced her to remain in bed at least 4 days out of the work week, rendering her unable to meet even the minimum requirements of her job. The illness also interfered with her social functioning in significant ways. For example, prior to the onset of chronic fatigue syndrome, Carmen had enjoyed going to dance clubs with her husband and friends on weekends. Although she had no history of marital difficulties prior to her illness and described her preillness relationship as loving and supportive, conflict with her husband began to occur more frequently as her health worsened and their income declined. Within a year, she found herself unemployed and separated. Carmen ultimately discovered that she had chronic fatigue syndrome after viewing a television program and seeking assessment and treatment from an immunologist specializing in chronic fatigue syndrome interviewed on the program. During subsequent years, Carmen's symptoms waxed and waned but never improved to the point where she was able to return to work. She tried a variety of recommended treatments and medications, including several types of antidepressants, some of which carried side effects that made her tremendously ill. Although some of the treatments she tried were effective in alleviating isolated symptoms (e.g., aspirin and acupuncture for headaches), they were not effective in terms of reducing the severity of her overall fatigue and eliminating most of her somatic symptoms.

The leader of a local chronic fatigue syndrome self-help group referred Carmen for assessment by a psychologist. The group leader recommended the assessment based upon the patient's disclosure of feelings of demoralization during a support group meeting. Because of Carmen's history of negative experiences with a variety of physicians who suggested that her illness was solely of psychiatric nature, she was initially reluctant to attend the assessment. Moreover, she had never consulted a psychologist before and did not know what to expect. However, the psychologist came highly recommended as an expert in CFS treatment, and Carmen decided to give the assessment a try because she felt she had nothing to lose.

## Assessment Phase

The ultimate goal of the initial interview is to obtain an empathic understanding of the presenting problems from the client's perspective. Feeling validated, understood, and having her experiences normalized would presumably increase Carmen's comfort with self-disclosure during the treatment process and increase the likelihood that she would be able to actively collaborate with the therapist in later identifying maladaptive beliefs and activity patterns. In addition to empathy, the therapist should carefully pace the interview by checking in with Carmen periodically to assess her reactions and energy levels in an effort to protect her from becoming so physically and emotionally overwhelmed that she would be reluctant to return for further treatment.

During the initial stage of assessment Carmen occasionally looked as if she were about to cry and had a great deal of difficulty with verbal and emotional expression. Upon exploring these difficulties further, Carmen explained that she did not feel comfortable discussing problems, thoughts, and feelings with a mental health professional because she feared that the professional might conclude that her illness was of purely psychiatric nature. She added that, prior to her illness, she had never felt she needed anyone's help or support because she had always served as a good listener and counselor for others. When asked about feelings of sadness, Carmen did acknowledge that she feels like she is in a "dark mood" approximately twice per week, particularly when her physical symptoms escalate and interfere with her day-to-day functioning. Recently, she has found it increasingly difficult to keep in touch with friends, and she has been grieving the loss of her husband. She added that these negative feelings first emerged approximately 3 months after the onset of chronic fatigue syndrome.

Carmen reported difficulty eating because she often suffers from gastrointestinal distress shortly after meals, and has lost approximately 20 pounds as a result. She reported that she feels particularly fatigued, nauseous, and dizzy after she wakes up in the morning, regardless of how much she slept the night before. On average, she either rests or sleeps approximately 16 hours per day. Lately, she has been reluctant to leave her home unless absolutely necessary because she fears she will become too tired or ill to make it back home using the public transportation system. As a result, she is feeling bored and isolated most of the time.

## Family History

Carmen is the youngest of four sisters. She was raised in a two-parent family in an urban, Mexican-American neighborhood. She described her parents as firm but nurturing and her older sisters as competitive but ultimately supportive. She described her community as a friendly, but dangerous, place to grow up. When asked to describe herself as a child, Carmen reported that she was well liked, intensely competitive, achievement oriented, and a talented and versatile athlete. She added that she also received guidance and mentoring from a maternal aunt, and two of her athletic coaches at school.

As evident from the beginning of the assessment phase, the assessment process began by meeting the client at whatever level of disclosure in which she was willing to engage. As the interview progressed, more specific questions were asked about the circumstances surrounding CFS onset, reactions of health care providers and individuals in Carmen's social network, illness-related losses, and issues involving self-concept and adaptation to illness. Ultimately, this process led to a discussion of emotional reactions and psychological symptoms.

Following the initial interview, a variety of assessment tools was employed to assess Carmen's functioning in the following areas: cognitive coping style, physical functioning, health care practices, social functioning, psychological functioning, and access to resources. Within the cognitive coping domain, the Fatigue-Related Cognitions Scale (Friedberg & Krupp, 1994) was used to provide a working map of symptom attribution and underlying beliefs that may influence Carmen's health care behaviors and emotional responses to the illness.

Within the domain of physical functioning, Carmen was encouraged to wear a pedometer (step counter) during predefined, 1-week periods at the beginning, middle, and end of the treatment process. In Carmen's case, the pedometer was used to measure changes in daily activity levels and compare physical functioning at the beginning, middle, and end of treatment. To accompany pedometer output, Carmen also completed a Daily Energy and Fatigue Record (Friedberg & Jason, in press) presented in Table 4 (p. 69) and in Appendix F (pp. 139–140). Using this record, Carmen provided daily ratings of her perceived and expended energy levels on a scale from 0 to 100 once daily in the evening before bed. In addition, Carmen rated the severity of her fatigue, dizziness, and nausea on a scale from 0 to 100 once in the morning after waking and once in the evening before bed. Carmen also provided ratings of positive and negative feelings from 0 to 100 once daily in the evening before bed. Finally, Carmen maintained a daily record of her sleep-wake activity and total hours of sleep per 24-hour period. Self-monitoring in these ways would facilitate Carmen's active engagement in the treatment process, and information generated provided insight into behavioral or emotional patterns that led to the worsening of her fatigue and CFS-related symptoms in the morning.

Within the health care practices domain, Carmen was assessed to have poor nutritional intake and was referred for consultation with a nutritionist. In addition, Carmen's use of drugs, alcohol, prescribed and over-the-counter medications, homeopathic remedies, vitamin

## Table 4: Summary of Treatment Goals With Psychometric and Activity Data

### Initial Treatment Goals

Improve my ability to think and remember things.

Decrease feelings of fatigue, particularly in the mornings, so one day I
might be able to return to work.

Decrease feelings of isolation.

### Psychometric Data

| | |
|---|---|
| Beck Anxiety Inventory | 9 |
| Beck Depression Inventory | 12 |
| Fatigue Severity Scale (Chalder et al., 1993) | 33 |

### Daily Energy and Fatigue Record (Friedberg & Jason, in press; Jason, Tryon, et al., 1997)*

| | Pedometer Ratings** (# Steps) | Perceived Energy (0-100) | Expended Energy (0-100) | Fatigue Severity (0-100) | Positive Feelings (0-100) | Negative Feelings (0-100) |
|---|---|---|---|---|---|---|
| Day 1 | 571 | 10 | 100 | 100 | 30 | 40 |
| Day 2 | 304 | 10 | 100 | 90 | 20 | 40 |
| Day 3 | 780 | 10 | 100 | 90 | 15 | 45 |
| Day 4 | 202 | 10 | 100 | 100 | 10 | 55 |
| Day 5 | 456 | 20 | 95 | 100 | 5 | 60 |
| Day 6 | 372 | 5 | 100 | 100 | 10 | 55 |
| Day 7 | 990 | 10 | 100 | 100 | 15 | 45 |

\* Ratings of perceived energy, expended energy, fatigue severity, positive feelings, and
negative feelings from 0 to 100, where 0 indicates the lowest rating for a particular
domain and 100 indicates the highest rating.

\*\* The patient's total number of walking steps was measured on a daily basis using an
electronic pedometer, which measures the number of steps taken based upon an individual's measured stride length. The patient wore the pedometer at all times for 7
consecutive days except when bathing and sleeping.

supplements, illicit drugs, and current daily caffeine intake was assessed. Carmen was also asked to describe her daily physical activity patterns in detail, and to identify any health-enhancing or self-soothing activities that she regularly practices or receives (e.g., massage, relaxation).

As part of the social support assessment, Carmen was asked if she regularly receives any physical forms of social support when ill (e.g., help with housecleaning, grocery shopping, errands, laundry, cooking). Assessment revealed that Carmen was not receiving assistance, so she was referred to a local independent living center to obtain low-cost personal assistance with daily chores and errands.

With respect to access to resources, a careful assessment of Carmen's access to health care and economic resources revealed that she had major medical insurance coverage and was receiving disability income.

## Identifying Goals and Reviewing Psychometric and Activity Data

The next phase of treatment involved identifying treatment goals and reviewing psychometric and activity data. Information regarding each of these components is presented in Table 4 (p. 69).

## Unique Features

One unique feature of this case involved complexities introduced by Carmen's medical condition, chronic fatigue syndrome. Fluctuations in energy levels, in the ability to process information, and in overall functional capabilities occasionally interfered with Carmen's ability to attend appointments regularly or sustain enough attention and concentration to remain actively engaged during a full 45-minute session. Thus, there was some allowance for last-minute rescheduling, no-charge cancellations, and shorter sessions, when needed. In addition, telephone therapy appointments were occasionally needed when Carmen was too ill to leave her home.

Another unique feature of this case involved Carmen's ethnic identification as Mexican-American. When relevant, issues pertaining to acculturation, use of language, and cultural beliefs about health and illness were considered in relation to treatment objectives. Furthermore, ethnocultural differences between the patient and therapist were also discussed when such differences became relevant within the therapeutic relationship.

## The Treatment Process

Treatment consisted of 16 sessions, each occurring once weekly with duration of 50 minutes in length. Three central objectives were important in socializing Carmen into cognitive-behavioral treatment using envelope theory. These included establishing empathy, planning for negative feelings within the therapeutic relationship, and outlining the essential elements of cognitive behavior therapy for the client. The most important of these objectives was to begin treatment by establishing a wholly empathic understanding of the presenting problems from the patient's perspective. Clear efforts toward empathic resonance demonstrated the therapist's willingness and openness to understand and work through the complexities and ambiguities of the CFS illness experience with Carmen. This approach increased Carmen's comfort with the treatment process and provided a corrective model for previous interactions with medical professionals (wherein Carmen felt stigmatized, inaccurately labeled, and invalidated).

In addition to maintaining an empathic response, the therapist worked hard to predict and manage effectively feelings of anger and negativity that arose within the treatment relationship. The therapist knew that any negative reactions Carmen had might have been attributable to a number of factors, including previous experiences of stigmatization and invalidation with other health care professionals, unavoidable breaks in empathy or "blind spots" in the therapist, and cultural inconsistencies between client and therapist. In preparing for these potential reactions, the therapist communicated to Carmen that the treatment process is collaborative in nature and that breaks in empathy or misunderstandings are necessary aspects of treatment that are bound to occur with attempts to identify and modify dysfunctional beliefs and behavior patterns. Together, Carmen and the therapist came up with a plan for managing situations involving negative interpersonal feelings, and the therapist asked Carmen to share her reactions with the therapist whenever she perceived breaks in empathy or misunderstandings between them.

In outlining the essential elements of cognitive behavior therapy, the therapist explained the relationship between events, beliefs, and behaviors to Carmen and emphasized the importance of the role of beliefs in influencing behavior. In addition, the therapist invited

Carmen to join her in collaboratively identifying and modifying her maladaptive beliefs or schemata and in altering dysfunctional behavior patterns.

Following the initial socialization phase, the therapist encouraged Carmen to assist her in constructing a treatment plan, listing three problems with corresponding objectives and goals. Using these goals, the therapist then began intervention using envelope theory as applied to cognitive behavior therapy. Carmen's Daily Energy and Fatigue Record in Table 4 (p. 69) indicated that she was not engaging in much physical activity (as evidenced by the low daily number of steps recorded on her pedometer ratings). In addition to her low level of functioning, Carmen documented very low levels of perceived energy resources (ranging from 5-20 on a scale of 100), but high levels of energy expenditure (ranging from 95-100 on a scale of 100). Given that Carmen seemed to have a very low level of perceived energy, but a high level of energy expenditure, application of the envelope theory first involved eliciting and identifying the beliefs that influenced Carmen to consistently overextend her energy resources through a process of Socratic questioning. For example, did Carmen feel compelled to overextend her energy resources in order to avoid negative judgment from herself or others? If Carmen did not push herself beyond her limitations, would it mean she was lazy or somehow inadequate? Did Carmen believe that overextending would not have a negative impact on her health status?

In addition to the identification of maladaptive beliefs that perpetuated overexertion, Carmen was asked to identify the specific behaviors and activities that demanded her highest energy output, and the circumstances under which she engaged in these activities were assessed. It was found that Carmen overengaged in exertion on days when she felt better than usual because she believed that she may have had to wait for a long period of time before she felt well enough to engage in the activity again. Carmen did not realize that, by overexerting herself on good days, she limited the overall number of good days that would ultimately be available to her. From a pragmatic standpoint, Carmen felt a strong obligation to continue to engage in activities that required high energy output, and her cognitions surrounding this felt obligation were not very flexible at first. Carmen was therefore encouraged to ask herself questions like "What would happen if I did not (engage in the high-energy activity) today?" "What would I really achieve by engaging in this activity today?" "What health consequences do I risk by engaging in this activity today?" Carmen was encouraged to carry out this cost-benefit analysis each time she considered engaging in activities that required energy expenditure and put her at risk for overexertion. After several sessions, Carmen's "must do" beliefs were modified, and she ultimately hired a low-cost, personal assistant to assist her with chores and errands. In addition, Carmen was more likely to elicit help and support from old friends. Now aware that CFS is a disability, she began to leave her home more often and take advantage of specialized public transportation services for the disabled. Carmen also took advantage of a home food delivery service, "Meals on Wheels," during periods of relapse.

Once Carmen began to experience an alleviation of fatigue and symptoms, she was urged to make a list of desired activities in order of priority in which the activities needed to be completed. She was then encouraged to rate each activity on the list from 0 to 100 in terms of the amount of energy she predicted it would require (with 0 indicating no energy required and 100 indicating maximum energy required). As she felt stronger, Carmen was encouraged to add activities slowly to her priority list over time and to make sure that she was aware of how much energy each activity required. This process of listing activities involved some reprioritizing and value reorientation, and Carmen quickly learned the value in designating restorative, self-soothing activities, such as meditation, breathing, relaxation, and gentle stretching exercises as high-priority activities. Such restorative activities carry a greater likelihood of leading to improvement in health status. Attempts to enlist social support and establish connection with supportive others who share similar interests and values were encouraged as other high-priority activities. For example, Carmen came to understand the value in replacing a solitary activity like housework with a restorative social activity, such as attending mass or an instructive seminar. In summary, Carmen was trained in the process of aggressive resting and positive mood enhancement. She began to realize the value of prioritizing activities carefully and of pacing herself using rest breaks and selective engagement when she was required to engage in prolonged exertion.

## Outcome

Given that Carmen had no history of psychiatric problems prior to becoming ill with CFS, and given that she did not appear to have any diagnosable character pathology, the outcome of psychotherapy was positive. Carmen learned to cope with her limitations more effectively, and she became more willing to leave her home and engage in social activity. Once Carmen attained a balance in perceived and expended energy, it was then possible to increase slowly the amount of activity that she engaged in. The key to her continued improvement was to not overexpend her energy supplies or consistently go outside her envelope.

# CHAPTER 7

# Cognitive-Behavioral Treatment II

This chapter focuses on cognitive and relaxation-oriented interventions. Although controversial illnesses may often be persistent and intractable, the styles of thinking, quality of mood, and level of distress experienced by these patients will determine their quality of life as much or more than the more salient dimensions of physical functioning and illness severity. Perhaps this is the challenge for the practitioner: to convince the client that, in the absence of substantial remission or recovery, quality of life can be significantly improved and maintained. This challenge is well illustrated in the following quotation from a 41-year-old man with CFS:

> As an exercise buff, I used to jog about 30 miles a week. When I developed the symptoms of CFS, I tried to ignore the symptoms and continue to exercise, but I finally collapsed from the abnormal fatigue that comes with the illness. I viewed stopping exercise as unacceptable, intolerable, and depressing. I didn't want to "cope," I wanted to be well. And I thought nothing short of being well would improve my sullen mood or pessimistic outlook. Then, after many months of unsuccessful doctor visits and ineffective treatments, I began to realize, through a combination of personal stress management, reading about the illness, and increased self-insight, that I could feel better emotionally. I hoped that these personal improvements might possibly help my physical symptoms, if not relieve them. I had to develop flexibility in the type of activities that I did, rather than be overinvolved with running. And I did find satisfaction in some low-level physical activity,

such as walking and golf (which I can handle in small doses, using a motorized cart to get from hole to hole). Before the illness I was too focused on work and exercise, to the exclusion of other things that I did not realize were so important to my well-being. I now recognize that balancing work and exercise with family and social involvements helps me physically as well as emotionally. CFS has been an important signal for me to change my lifestyle to be more balanced and flexible. Does that mean that the illness has been a good thing? Of course not. But by prioritizing goals with my health in mind, I have seen a tremendous benefit. I'm not totally well, but I'm about 70% back to normal.

## The Interactive Symptom-Stress Model

According to the interactive symptom-stress model, the fundamental mechanism of stress creation in controversial illnesses involves three steps: (a) Initially, illness symptoms and limitations trigger negative emotions such as discouragement, depression, anxiety, and anger; (b) these emotions generate more fatigue, pain, and other somatic symptoms; and (c) these increased illness symptoms, in turn, intensify the negative emotions. Thus, an interactive cycle of symptoms and reactive stress is initiated and maintained. The negative emotions are associated with maladaptive cognitive coping strategies and dysfunctional thoughts. It should be noted that negative emotions may, in part, contribute to the development of these illnesses and may also be a reactive byproduct of them. Cognitive and behavioral interventions may be helpful for both types of emotional distress.

Many patients are not at all aware of the effect of persistent, low-level emotional stress on their symptoms and well-being. Conversely, some are not aware of the effects of their symptoms on their overall emotional well-being, and it may often take others to make them aware of their changes in mood and frustration tolerance. These stress factors arise from the ordinary events of daily living, such as work, housekeeping, childcare, and marital interactions. Because it is difficult for patients to recognize the negative effects of these stressors, increased symptoms are thought to be solely the result of unpredictable fluctuations in the illness. Yet emotional stress will meld imperceptibly into the illness experience and result in greater symptom intensity. Thus, patients may not accept the usefulness of cognitive or relaxation interventions because they cannot identify the important contribution of stress to the severity of their illness.

The techniques described next are designed to make patients aware of stress contributions to their illness and to show them how to interrupt and diffuse the escalating cycle of stress-symptom interactions. These clinical interventions, including relaxation training, imaginal desensitization, pleasant mood induction, cognitive coping skills, activity pacing, social support enhancement, and memory assistance, are generally applicable to CFS, FMS, and MCS. If a particular technique has special relevance to one of these illnesses, it will be noted.

## Relaxation Training

Given the high levels of emotional distress that these patients initially present, the most immediately useful and beneficial technique may be deep relaxation. In addition to reducing emotional and physical stress, relaxation can improve well-being, reduce illness symptoms (including FMS-related pain), lessen muscular tension, serve as a coping skill, and improve mental clarity. Relaxation training is especially useful when the patient's physical and emotional distress is not appreciably reduced via supportive therapeutic dialogue or cognitive coping techniques. Specific relaxation scripts that can be used by the psychotherapist are printed below.

### Script One: Breathing Focus

Breathing can serve as an excellent means of relaxation, carrying added benefits of increasing oxygenation to the blood, strengthening respiratory muscles (especially the diaphragm), and cleansing the lungs of stale air. The following is a script* that combines breathing focus and relaxation:

> One, let your eyes close. Two, take a long, deep breath, and three, slowly release the breath. Feel the release, the letting go as you exhale and allow your breathing to assume an easy, natural rhythm. Focus on the easy breathing rhythm . . . inhale and exhale. Simply observe it and recognize it as a natural process, an easy response and a source of relaxation. . . . Observation is simply passive attention to your own natural rhythms.

*Note. From *Coping With Chronic Fatigue Syndrome: Nine Things You Can Do* (pp. 67–68), by F. Friedberg, 1995, Oakland, CA: New Harbinger. Copyright © 1995 by New Harbinger. Reprinted with permission.

Appreciate them. . . . Now focus on the release of breath. Each time you exhale, you release tension as well as breath. With each exhale, there is a perceptible release of tension, as well as breath. Exhale, release; exhale, release. . . . Feel the release, the letting go that accompanies each release of breath. Exhale, release. . . . Now allowing relaxed feelings to radiate upward to the shoulders, going across the shoulders and descending through both arms. Upper arms relaxed . . . lower arms relaxed . . . both arms relaxing. Now relaxed feelings descending through the chest, flowing into the stomach, the stomach becoming relaxed. Relaxed sensations spreading through the hips and to the upper legs and enveloping the upper legs. Now flowing to the lower legs . . . all the way down to the feet. The feet becoming loose and relaxed, loose and relaxed. Relaxed sensations retracing their gentle path upward. Lower legs relaxed . . . upper legs relaxed. Relaxed feelings ascending the lower back, lower back loosening. . . . Now proceeding to the upper back . . . up the back of the neck . . . infusing the area with relaxed sensations. Now spreading up over the scalp and down the face . . . forehead relaxed, eyes relaxed, jaw becoming loose, limp, and slack; loose, limp, and slack.

You have reached a pleasant plateau of calm and comfort. Recognize the feelings you now have. Know that you can reproduce these feelings with regular easy practice. . . . Now, as I count from one to ten, you can feel even more relaxed: 1, more relaxed; 2, even more; 3, deeper down; 4, more relaxed; 5, calmer still; 6, even more; 7, deeper down; 8, more relaxed; 9, so very calm; 10, your entire physical self completely immersed in relaxed sensations . . . calm, wavy deep relaxation, so deeply and comfortably relaxed.

Now refocus on the easy breathing rhythm, the source of profound release and relaxation. As you inhale, say to yourself, reee. . . . And as you exhale, laaax. . . . A long reee as you inhale and a slow laax as you exhale. Ree. . . . Laax. Now I'd like you to take the next minute to say the re-lax phrase to yourself along with your breathing. Go ahead now and my voice will return shortly. (Pause for one minute.)

All right. Very good. Continue relaxing and recognize the feelings you now have at this deeper level. Recognize your ability to reproduce these feelings with regular easy practice.

Now, when it is comfortable for you, slowly open your eyes, bringing yourself back to wakefulness; feeling relaxed and refreshed.

## Pleasant Imagery

Some clients prefer a relaxation technique that focuses on such pleasant imagery as the beach, the country, or the mountains. Such visualizations may be more effective for clients who experience "racing" thoughts and an inability directly to relax their thinking with body-focused techniques, such as breathing focus. These clients may better respond to the distraction provided by imagined pleasant scenes. Although these techniques may be as effective as breathing focus, the breathing method has the advantage of "portability." It can be used quickly and easily as a coping skill in many situations.

If the patient has difficulty relaxing with breathing focus, or would like to enhance his or her relaxation experience, the transcript* below of a beach scene can also be incorporated into the therapy session or recorded as a taped exercise.

Imagine yourself spending an afternoon at the beach. The sand feels warm and soft against your skin. You are sitting on the sand observing the ocean, the azure blue water; viewing the flow of the waves as they move rhythmically to the shore, the water becoming a light transparent green as it flows to the shoreline. And you see the whitecaps on the waves as the waves roll onto the shore; yes, waves gently reaching the shore, like sparkling water spilling on the sand; feeling a salty, refreshing spray in the air, that refreshing misty spray permeating your body — so wonderfully invigorating and uplifting; revitalizing and relaxing.

Allow yourself the next few moments to imagine the pleasant flow of the waves onto the shore as they rise and fall, rise and fall. Go ahead now and imagine the waves. (Pause for about 5 seconds.)

All right. Very good. Now you decide to take an easy stroll along the beach as you view the surf; yes, observe the curving shoreline off in the distance, the curving shoreline as it merges

---

*__Note.__ From *Coping With Chronic Fatigue Syndrome: Nine Things You Can Do* (pp. 58-59), by F. Friedberg, 1995, Oakland, CA: New Harbinger. Copyright © 1995 by New Harbinger. Reprinted with permission.

with the horizon. As you walk onward, onward, you feel the sand crunching beneath your feet; such a pleasant sensation — the warm crunchy sand. It complements the warmth of the sun overhead. Feel the warmth of the sun on your back, that gentle warmth flowing down your back and throughout your body; comfortable warmth from the sun filling you with pleasant sensations. With your senses so very aware, you notice the sand dunes rising along the beach, sand dunes with isolated clumps of tall grass on their slopes. Noticing the tall grass gently swaying in the breeze. The breezes creating tranquil feelings.

And as you walk onward, you hear the sound of seagulls in the distance. A flock of white seagulls approaching, flying so easily, gliding in the wind, making their distinctive sounds passing overhead. Now flying off in the distance, leaving you with a feeling of serenity. . . . Now feeling a gentle breeze at your back. The gentle breeze coaxing you further along, heightening your senses.

As you look across the waves, you see a sleek white sailboat moving through the water. The boat moving so gracefully, the sails filled with gently sweeping winds. Enjoy the silent steadiness of the boat as it moves along with the wind.

Now as you gaze further toward the horizon, you see the sun setting. Yes, the sun setting in a full display of vivid colors: bright yellows, deep reds, and burnt oranges against the light gray clouds and a pale blue sky. As the sun descends, it projects a long wedge of yellow light across the water; slowly sinking down. And a breathtaking serenity begins to pervade the atmosphere. An emerging serenity so deep that it is fully absorbing your senses.

Now you begin to conclude the experience — finish the experience with acceptance and peace, acceptance and peace . . . . Allow yourself the next minute, all the time in the world, all the time you need to bring yourself back to wakefulness, your eyes opening slowly, feeling relaxed and refreshed.

## Healing Imagery

Despite the extensive media coverage on mind/body cures, there is no convincing evidence that relaxation or healing imagery will cure CFS or other chronic illnesses such as cancer or heart disease.

However, healing imagery can be a constructive way to "fight" the illness, and generate hope. Thus it can be a useful alternative or addition to standard relaxation techniques. The transcript* below incorporates healing suggestions:

> Your healing can now begin, yes, your healing begins from within yourself. An inner radiance that begins as a mere speck of light, yes, an inner point of light and warmth . . . radiating strength and power . . . yes, the strength and power that grows warm and radiant . . . inner strength. Feel it, experience it fully, thoroughly, inner radiance growing stronger. . . . Ready now, yes ready to direct its healing strength towards your weakened system. Yes, the inner radiance directing its strength towards your body. Feel that inner sense of strength beginning, working within your body. Feeling revitalized, re-energize . . . strengthening as your inner radiance strengthens and energizes. Feel the warm, intense energy doing its work; reactivating, restoring your body . . . yes, restoring your body. Experience that strengthening fully, thoroughly, that inner boosting, growing even stronger now, stronger, more powerful than before. And as you feel that strength, you believe in yourself and your ability to succeed in your goal of rebuilding your body. Yes, believing in the strength of your thoughts, images, and the totality of your internal powers. You believe so strongly, feeling that boost even now, yes, yet remaining tolerant, letting time pass, knowing that any worthwhile goal takes time, any worthwhile goal. And you have resolved to accomplish your goal, believing you can . . . re-energizing, boosting your system. You hold firmly to that belief; yes, so firmly . . . feeling less fatigued . . . and this message remains with you, far beyond these words, far beyond these words. Now, slowly bringing yourself back to wakefulness, eyes opening gradually, feeling relaxed and refreshed.

Generally, we will teach one of these relaxation techniques, usually the breathing-focus relaxation method, during the first or second visit, and prescribe it for home use. The patient is told to practice the "re-lax" phrase for 10 minutes in the a.m and 10 minutes in the

---

*Note. From *Coping With Chronic Fatigue Syndrome: Nine Things You Can Do* (pp. 70-71), by F. Friedberg, 1995, Oakland, CA: New Harbinger. Copyright © 1995 by New Harbinger. Reprinted with permission.

p.m. before meals and in a quiet setting without distractions or inter-ruptions. If the patient has trouble falling or staying asleep, it is also assigned as a sleep-induction technique before bedtime. Usually, the individual obtains some benefit from the breathing technique. However, a more profound feeling of relaxation may be achieved when they are guided by an audiotape. Thus, after the initial week of self-guided relaxation, we provide clients with a relaxation tape based on one or more of the preceding relaxation scripts as recorded by the ther-apist. Because the relaxation tape reinforces the association between deep relaxation and the re-lax phrase, significant relaxation without the tape can then be generated in only a minute or 2 using the breath-ing focus method. The re-lax phrase is also a portable relaxation method that can be used almost anywhere as a stress-reduction and relaxation technique.

In addition to its calming effects, the tape may be helpful in coun-teracting patients' resistance to relaxation, which they may consider to be a waste of time. Even for those who are too disabled to do major physical activities, mental planning may seem more productive than taking time to do "nothing" and relax. With their attention focused on a tape, patients are better able to distract from their own action-oriented thoughts and understand through personal experience how relaxation can improve their physical and emotional well-being. Re-sistance to relaxation may also be reduced by coping self-statements such as "I have the right to take time for myself"; or "relaxation will help me feel better and be more efficient."

## Imaginal Desensitization in MCS

In the case of MCS, symptomatic reactions to low level chemical exposures may generate significant stress. Some patients become so emotionally traumatized by their symptoms that even the thought of a particular chemical exposure is enough to provoke a stress reaction or an MCS symptomatic response. In such cases, cognitive and relax-ation techniques can be applied to assist individuals in coping with their symptoms as they encounter them.

One potential means of facilitating coping is for the therapist and patient initially to construct a hierarchy of chemical exposures, rang-ing from the least to the most provocative. (Toxic exposures commonly reported in MCS include shower curtains, new carpeting, pesticides, auto exhaust, and tobacco smoke.) Next, the therapist relaxes the client with a standard relaxation procedure. Then, the therapist asks the patient to imagine being exposed to the lowest item on the hierarchy. If any type of symptomatic reaction is reported, the client is given relaxation suggestions until the reaction subsides, with the added instruction to use such procedures in order to cope in the event of an actual exposure. The same item is then visualized once again and followed by relaxation procedures until no response is elicited. The same procedure is followed for the next item on the hierarchy until all the items on the list have been covered. As a result of this procedure, the patient then learns the power of relaxation as applied to a stressful symptomatic situation, such as a chemical exposure.

Although this procedure has been evaluated only in two case studies, it is likely to produce a potentially significant reduction in stress reactions to symptoms, particularly when the therapist and patient are willing to accept the notion that these procedures are designed to improve coping and lessen stressful reactions, rather than "cure" the conditions themselves.

## Pleasant Mood Induction

Recent empirical evidence as well as clinical observation of CFS patients indicates that generating pleasant mood will reduce distress, ameliorate somatic symptoms, and even improve functioning, although perhaps only temporarily. Pleasant mood that is maintained over an extended period of time may also indicate a healthy realignment of life priorities. Clinical treatment of patients with FMS and MCS suggests that pleasant mood may have similar salutary effects. However, mood elevation is difficult when one is chronically ill. And it may be an even greater challenge for those with controversial illnesses who carry the additional burdens of others' skepticism, lower levels of social support, and, for those patients with comorbid depression, poor tolerance of standard doses of antidepressant medication. Despite these obstacles, the technique of pleasant mood induction can still be a valuable and effective tool for the psychotherapist in treating these patients, and patients generally respond positively to implementation of this aspect of the intervention.

Because ongoing stress and lifestyle disruptions often dominate the lives of people with controversial illnesses, the potential benefit of creating pleasant experiences may be deemphasized or disregarded entirely in their daily living. To introduce pleasant mood induction, the clinician should point out to clients that integrating small but positive events and experiences into their daily lives can uplift mood and allow intrusive symptoms to recede. Examples of low effort activities include listening to an inspirational speaker, sharing a special moment with a friend, watching ducks on a pond, reading an entertaining short story, experiencing autumn foliage, and so forth. The therapist can guide the client toward these simple endeavors with the incentive that such activities will yield a powerful and perhaps enduring therapeutic benefit.

## Cognitive Coping Skills

Our approach to cognitive coping is based on the principles of rational-emotive behavior therapy (Ellis, 1997). Initially, we help the patient to identify the damaging beliefs that increase illness severity, create stress, and heighten frustration toward the illness, the self, and the environment. One category of damaging beliefs, discomfort intolerance, derives from the patient's intolerance of his or her symptoms, functional limitations, and lifestyle disruptions. Discomfort intolerance may be expressed in anger-producing thoughts such as "I should be able to control this illness!"; "I hate being limited from what I want to do!"; and "I can't stand my life the way it is!" It is important to point out to the patient how the stress generated by these beliefs will cause further deterioration in quality of life and that the reduction of this stress can restore some sense of control. With this goal of stress reduction in mind, the patient's damaging beliefs can be constructively challenged. For instance, we might ask the patient, "Why should you be able to control this illness? Where is the evidence?" The client can be shown that such "control" beliefs are based on personal rules of behavior that may not apply when one has a chronic illness.

It can be explained to clients that the strong desire to control and subdue the illness does not mean that they should or must be able to exert such control. Such demands for illness control, although understandable, can produce sustained upset. Thus, it is stress reducing for the client to learn to endure and tolerate limitations rather than rail against them. As the patient's erroneous ideas about total self-control over his or her illness are effectively disputed, the realization can evolve that a life of good health and vitality, uninterrupted by persistent conditions is, unfortunately, more of a cultural myth than an established reality for a large percentage of the population. Despite this unfortunate reality, a good quality of life can be attained by those with chronic illnesses.

Anger may also be directed at spouses, adult children, or close friends because they do not offer the physical and emotional support that the patient expects. Because anger, in its many manifestations, may be a prominent feature of the clinical presentation, the therapist should help the patient to identify angry feelings and reinforce the patient's right to experience and express anger. Appropriate assertive behavior should be taught and modeled in session for subsequent use with significant others. Some patients may believe that it is unacceptable to be angry or to express anger openly because their complaints may not be justified. The threat of disapproval from significant others and its effect on self-esteem can be managed by assigning coping statements that the patient practices at home. Examples of coping statements are "My partner's annoyance with me does not make me a bad person" and "Although I would like my partner's approval, I am not diminished as a person if I don't get it." Finally, as the patient becomes more assertive and effective with significant others, the anger-producing demand that others *must* be more supportive and helpful can be challenged with coping statements such as "There is no rule that my 'significant other' must or should be more helpful. I will do what I can to ask for help. If I get it, fine. If not, that is unfortunate, not terrible."

Discouragement is another emotion commonly seen in controversial illnesses. Discouragement is the understandable result of the limitations created by these chronic conditions. However, discouragement can lead to an unhealthy dwelling on illness symptoms with thoughts such as "I'm so sick. I'm so sick." The therapist can explain how dwelling on such illness thoughts leads to persistently low feelings and pessimism. The patient can then learn to reduce focusing on these thoughts by first identifying the dwelling process when it occurs and then by cognitively distracting to other activities. It is better for the client to be (appropriately) disappointed about limitations, rather than to escalate feelings of disappointment into a preoccupation with negative illness thoughts.

Guilt about not carrying out personal and family responsibilities is yet another reactive emotion experienced by those with controversial illnesses. This emotion is based on the damaging belief that one should be able to do all that one wants for others despite illness limitations. This inability to help and care for others to the degree that was done prior to being ill becomes equated with being inadequate, weak, or useless. Such self-diminishing thoughts can be challenged by pointing out to the client that self-labeling is an inaccurate overgeneralization about the self. According to the theory of rational therapy, one can rate or judge his or her specific actions but cannot accurately rate the entire self. So the patient can be taught to limit guilt-producing self-condemnation by avoiding self-rating and, instead, feeling (appropriately) sorry about things that he or she cannot do for others. In this way, the patient learns to separate his or her sense of self from the illness.

### Coping With Disbelief

For those whose illnesses are maligned, dismissed, and even ridiculed, the problem of professional and public disbelief may become an important coping issue. Patients confronted with disbelieving others may react with anger and defensiveness based on beliefs such as "I should be believed!" and "Can't they see how sick I am?" As a result, people with controversial illnesses may decide to visit a psychotherapist in order to receive interpersonal validation of their illness concerns. Above all else, the therapist should offer unconditional support for the client's symptom presentation as well as understanding of the emotional stress generated by the illness. Coping statements for the patient that can be useful in moderating the stress triggered by disbelief include (a) "I cannot convince anyone that I am ill who does not want to believe it"; (b) "Others' disbelief does not negate the reality of my illness"; and (c) "People are uncomfortable with others who have disabling illnesses and may try to minimize my illness so they feel less vulnerable to such a threat." The patient can also learn to respond in a more constructive way to those who express disbelief. For instance, changing the subject may be a better alternative than continuing a useless argument about the existence of the patient's illness. Or if the skeptic offers shopworn advice about ready cures, home remedies, and new miracle treatments, the patient can respond that he or she will "think about it." This vague answer leaves the advice giver nowhere to go except, hopefully, to a different subject.

## Activity Pacing

Activity pacing involves moderating activity and behavior so that it does not fall into the extremes of overexertion and collapse — a pattern often reported by patients with CFS, FMS, and MCS. The overwork-collapse pattern is, to a large extent, maintained by the symptom of postexertional malaise wherein minimal exertion can sometimes lead to substantial and disabling symptom flare-ups. Initial evidence for the overwork-collapse pattern has been found in patients with CFS, and may also be applied to those with FMS. The findings of a study by Friedberg (2000) revealed that high levels of physical activity, as measured by a step-counter during a particular day, predicted significantly lower levels of activity the next day, thus confirming an up-and-down pattern for about half of the study participants. Although the down period could not be characterized by collapse, it was clear that these patients were reacting with lower activity and increased symptoms the day after feeling better and doing more.

It is helpful to ask the client to keep a record of his or her activities and symptoms (see Appendix F on pages 139–140 for a record form; Friedberg & Jason, in press) for a 1- or 2-week period in order to see if such a behavioral pattern is present and how it may be affecting his or her symptoms and well-being. For example, when a patient is feeling physically better, he or she may follow a preillness schedule of compulsively finishing a number of tasks with no flexibility for reducing activity if symptoms begin to flare. Based on a review of the activity record, the therapist can discuss with the client how activity can be moderated. It is often difficult to influence clients to alter their routines from the typical up-and-down patterns to a more healthy moderated schedule, yet even small changes in these behavioral extremes may lead to important and healthy lifestyle adjustments. Once identified, the patient's ability to cut back voluntarily on potentially damaging overactivity is an important component of an activity pacing strategy.

### Exposure Avoidance Treatment in MCS

A principal treatment modality for MCS involves minimizing exposure to the offending chemicals using such tactics as eliminating carpeting, pesticides, and cleaning agents from the home and avoiding perfume, tobacco smoke, and other substances experienced as toxic (Lawson, 1993). Avoidance may also include consuming chemical-free food and water; wearing nonsynthetic clothing free of pesticides and formaldehyde; living in housing with good ventilation, air purifiers, and no toxic paint, carpeting, or synthetic furniture; and restriction of travel in areas where avoidance is possible (Davis et al., 1998). If avoidance is achieved and individuals with MCS live in safe housing, it is possible that they will be able to improve and function at a level close to their original baseline. In a survey of treatments used by individuals with MCS, 41% of whom also had CFS (LeRoy et al.,

1996), 93% were helped by chemical avoidance, and 86% were helped by creating environmentally safe homes. In a study by Davis et al. (1998), MCS participants were divided into two separate groups, those who reported living in safe housing and those who reported living in unsafe housing. Individuals with MCS who lived in environmentally safe housing were significantly less disabled by MCS-related symptoms.

## Social Support

Received social support can lessen the burden of these illnesses. Such support involves others helping the patient with physical tasks and offering empathy for emotional distress. Perhaps there is an optimal level of social support that is beneficial for people with controversial illnesses. If physical and emotional support are lacking, the patient may suffer health-compromising stress as a result of taxing limited physical capacities. At the other extreme, too much social support, which might take the form of overprotectiveness by a spouse, may leave the patient feeling more disabled than necessary. The optimal level of social support is not a fixed entity but is determined by the patient's level of energy, pain, and general symptom severity at any particular time. Appropriate levels of physical and emotional support allow the patient to feel as functional as possible yet allow time for rest and recuperation when symptoms are overwhelming. The specifics of how much support is needed are best negotiated with the spouse or other caregiver in frank and open discussions. It should be noted that the healthy spouse also has important needs that are often neglected due to the illness of his or her partner. Indeed, the healthy spouse has the right to negotiate for the things he or she wants from the ill partner in order to maintain a satisfactory relationship. If one partner is unable to engage the other in a productive discussion about support or reciprocity in the relationship, then a marital therapist who specializes in chronic illnesses may be desirable.

An additional means of social support may be provided through local and national self-help group organizations, such as the CFIDS Association of America. Such groups can provide a wide variety of support, ranging from educational information about the illnesses to emotion-based coping. Appendix G (pp. 141–145) contains a list of self-help group organizations and other useful resources for clinicians and patients with these conditions. While some professionals may feel that support groups may serve to prolong and reinforce illness behavior, research suggests that self-initiated forms of treatment that foster empowerment, rather than dependency on the medical system, can facilitate goal setting and contribute to improvements in overall quality of life.

## Memory Assistance

Cognitive difficulties are reported by the great majority of individuals with CFS, FMS, and MCS. These difficulties include attention, concentration, and short-term memory problems. Patients may have trouble remembering routine information, difficulty focusing on conversations, or finding the right word. Any distraction from their immediate focus of attention may derail their thinking.

Several practical suggestions may be helpful to cope with these cognitive problems, including the use of such memory aids as appointment books, calendar notes, and post-its. Second, organizing the day into manageable units of cognitive activity, rather than forcing sustained mental effort, is also helpful. Third, doing one thing at a time is less disruptive to cognitive processes than multiple tasking. For instance, balancing a checkbook while listening to the radio may produce cognitive overload. Because rapid mental fatigue is associated with cognitive difficulties in these illnesses, relaxation breaks to restore mental energy may also be useful. Patients can also be made aware of recent research findings providing evidence for decreased cognitive functioning with physical overexertion. Using this paradigm, they may be able to predict cognitive symptom increases associated with overexertion.

## Case Example of CFS Treatment

The case of Nancy, the individual with CFS presented in Chapter 3, revealed potentially modifiable traits that were related to a behavioral pattern of overwork and collapse. During the course of five cognitive-behavioral treatment sessions over 2 months, Nancy learned to pace her activity and recognized the early premonitory signals of symptomatic flare-ups and behavioral collapse. One form of activity pacing involved cleaning her house in small increments rather than in one massive, uninterrupted effort. She also experimented with new nonharried behaviors such as leaving a low level of disarray in her house, like an unmade bed for several days. Although this conscious lack of attention to housekeeping raised her anxiety level by preventing a compulsive response, she learned to counteract the irrational thinking that everything must be in order at all times. In her words, "It will eventually get done."

Her belief that she could not decline social invitations was another target for cognitive restructuring of a health-damaging belief. She used the cognitive coping statement that she *could* tolerate her friends' (presumed) disapproval if she declined an invitation or if she left them early due to increasing fatigue symptoms (an early signal was stiffness in the back of her neck). By the end of treatment, she reported significant reductions in CFS and stress symptoms and reduced downtime, from 1 to 2 weeks a month to only 3 or 4 days per month. In addition, relaxation training helped to (a) reinforce a healthier lifestyle of moderated activity, (b) generate feelings of well-being, and (c) reduce fatigue. Now she could better distinguish between normal tiredness and the abnormal fatigue associated with CFS. As a result, she could adjust her activities accordingly so as to minimize fatigue flare-ups.

## Case Example of FMS Treatment

The case of Alison (presented in Chapter 3) well illustrates the symptoms associated with FMS, including generalized bodily pain, fatigue, sleep disturbance, and migraine headache. The patient's reluctance to reduce her illness-exacerbating workload and to ask for much needed support are associated psychological features of the illness in many patients. Over the course of several visits, she identified the core philosophical beliefs that were driving her symptom-exacerbating behaviors. These beliefs included (a) "If I can't handle all of my responsibilities, I'm weak and people will not like me"; (b) "I have no right to complain or ask for support because my life should be very fulfilling with a good husband, children, and a good job"; and (c) "I must be active and productive at all times, otherwise I am indolent and lazy." In a behavioral intervention designed to dispute these damaging beliefs, she accepted an invitation to a church-sponsored excursion to Colorado, which entailed a few leisurely meetings with considerable time for rest and relaxation. The vacation acted as a vehicle for her to reevaluate her overwhelming responsibilities and to take specific actions to reduce this excessive level of obligation.

After the trip, she began to play her guitar for 30 minutes a day and enjoyed the soothing experience. In addition, she used prescribed relaxation techniques to hasten sleep onset and get a more restful night's sleep. Alison also devised stress-reducing alternatives to her responsibilities with her kids. Rather than taking them to all of their afterschool activities, she arranged for car pooling with other parents, which gave her more personal time. She now began to recognize that leisure time was an important and healthy behavior, rather than an unnecessary personal indulgence. Over several weeks, her FMS symptoms lessened from their most severe levels; however, her teaching job continued to trigger symptom flare-ups. A reevaluation of her perceived obligation to remain on the job now became an important focus of her attention. Finally, she asked for (and received) more physical support from her husband as well as greater levels of one-on-one interaction which had been lacking for many years. Although her FMS symptoms substantially lessened, she still experienced bodily pain and, therefore, was not in remission or recovery. Yet this was a highly favorable outcome for a cognitive-behavioral intervention in FMS — an illness that is often refractory to medical treatment.

## Case Example of MCS Treatment

The case of Carolyn described in Chapter 3 was a challenging one for her clinician who was presented with both generalized anxiety disorder and disabling MCS. Once situated in safe housing in a relatively pollution-free area of the country, the patient's continued high level of mental and emotional arousal, expressed as chronic anxiety, worry, irritability, and anger suggested the utility of relaxation training to reduce her distress and generate a sense of emotional self-control and well-being. Relaxation training did indeed reduce her high levels of emotional distress. Also, she benefited from leisurely outdoor walks, which allowed her to challenge her fears and partially counteract her negative emotional reactions to the illness and its limitations. Furthermore, she designed a daily schedule of house maintenance, light reading, and care of her daughter. This daily activity structuring brought some order into her life that had been so dominated by MCS and anxiety symptoms. Finally, she effectively used cognitive coping techniques to promote self-tolerance of her emotional reactivity rather than angry intolerance and self-rejection due to her emotional "weakness." Despite these achievements, given the severity of her symptoms, Carolyn had great difficulty maintaining emotional control and sometimes had highly charged conflicts with her husband over the deterioration of their relationship. Therefore, a trial of antianxiety medication was recommended.

Despite her chemical sensitivity, Carolyn was able to tolerate and benefit from a course of low dosage Klonopin, which reduced some of her ongoing anxiety. Although unable to resume working, she used the relaxation techniques, cognitive and behavioral coping skills, daily structuring of activities, and avoidance of particular chemical exposures which, in combination, improved her quality of life.

# CHAPTER 8

# Summary and Future Directions

Chronic fatigue syndrome (CFS), fibromyalgia (FMS), and multiple chemical sensitivities (MCS) are debilitating illnesses that affect significant portions of the U.S. population. These conditions often impact all aspects of life functioning, including employment and activities of daily living. Appropriate assessment and treatment of these conditions are characterized by multiple layers of complexity and often involve a high need for integrative planning and comprehensive service implementation. To date, effective, affordable, comprehensive assessment and treatment programs do not exist to address both the medical and social service needs of individuals with these illnesses. Thus, future planning to treat these populations should focus on the development of such a program where individuals can be individually assessed and where treatment can be specifically tailored to meet the unique needs of the patients. Ultimately, the program would enhance the welfare of individuals with these conditions both directly, through the delivery of services, and indirectly, through public education and the increased allocation of resources. There is a significant need to develop model programs that can ultimately be disseminated to those individuals who need these services.

The program would provide a thorough and individualized assessment, which would lead to access to medical and social services provided by practitioners that are specialized in the areas of CFS, FMS, and MCS. A comprehensive treatment plan would be developed for each client based on that individual's need. This might include focusing on increasing physical, social, psychological, and/or occupational functioning. The program would also provide resources to educate clients and their families about these conditions. Based on individual needs, the program would link clients with needed assistance such as financial assistance, housing, and activities of daily living. Emphasis will be placed on providing clients with a support network of similar others and with service providers. Patients would therefore be empowered by actively participating in the identification of what is offered in the comprehensive center. Services available through the program would be developed through the collaboration of on-site and local health and social service professionals and in conjunction with experts in the area of CFS, FMS, and MCS. Guidance would also be provided through local and national CFS, FMS, and MCS self-help organizations.

The program would also provide advocacy services, including educating the public, particularly medical and vocational service providers, about the nature and treatment of these conditions, and about the services offered by the program. The program would work toward social policy change at a larger level, increasing the provision of effective services and resources by utilizing the voices of patients and professionals working together. These efforts would increase acceptance and acknowledgment of these conditions, and the public, both general and medical, would become more responsive to the needs of individuals with these disabling conditions.

# Table of Contents

# Chronic Fatigue Syndrome Self-Report Questionnaire

1.  a.  Are you currently experiencing any problems with fatigue or tiredness (check one)?

    ❏ No    ❏ Yes

    b.  *If you replied "Yes" to 1a,* when did the fatigue begin?

    _____

2.  When your problem with fatigue began, did it develop (check one):

    ❏ Rapidly–within 24 hours
    ❏ Over 1 week        ❏ Over 1 month
    ❏ Over 2-6 months    ❏ Over 7-12 months
    ❏ Over 1-2 years     ❏ Longer than 2 years
    ❏ Had problems with fatigue since childhood or adolescence
    ❏ N/A–Not having a problem with fatigue

3.  In the past month, how many hours a week have you spent doing

    household related activities?    _____
    social-related activities?       _____
    work-related activities?         _____

4.  a.  In the past 6 months, have you had to reduce the number of hours you previously spent on occupational, social, or family activities because of your health problems with fatigue (check one)?

    ❏ No    ❏ Yes

b.   *If you replied "Yes" to 4a,* which activities and by how many hours per week have you cut back?

Occupational:   Decreased by ___ hours/week
Social:         Decreased by ___ hours/week
Family:         Decreased by ___ hours/week

c.   *If you replied "Yes" to 4a,* how many hours did you use to spend on

Occupational activities?   _____
Social activities?         _____
Family activities?         _____

5. a.   If you rest, does your fatigue go away entirely, partially, or does rest have no effect on your fatigue (check one)?

❏ Entirely    ❏ Partially    ❏ No effect

b.   *If you replied "Entirely" or "Partially" to 5a:*

How long do you have to rest before your fatigue entirely or partially goes away?_____
Will your fatigue return if you stop resting and start doing something (check one)?        ❏ No    ❏ Yes

6. Do you restrict your activity levels to avoid experiencing severe fatigue (check one)?

❏ No    ❏ Yes

7. How does physical activity make you feel (check one)?

❏ Worse    ❏ Better    ❏ Has no effect

8. a.   In the past 6 months, how often have you experienced a persistent or recurrent problem with postexertional malaise (check one)? By postexertional malaise I mean do you begin to feel worse after engaging in activities that require either physical or mental exertion?

❏ Never            ❏ Seldom
❏ Often or Usually ❏ Always

b.   *If you replied "Often or Usually" or "Always" to 8a,* how long does the postexertional malaise last (check one)?

❏ Less than 1 hour
❏ 1-3 hours

☐ 4-10 hours
☐ 11-13 hours
☐ More than 13 hours _____ (specify how long)
☐ More than 24 hours

c. *If you replied "Never" or "Seldom" to 8a,* what about if you exercise—Do you experience increased fatigue or a worsening of your symptoms after engaging in exercise (check one)?

☐ No ☐ Yes

d. *If you replied "No" to 8c,* is that because you are not exercising, or does exertion just not affect your symptoms, or does it even make you feel better (check one)?

☐ Not exercising ☐ No effect ☐ Feel better

e. *If you replied "Not Exercising" to 8d,* why aren't you exercising (check one)?

☐ Not interested
☐ No time
☐ Would like to but cannot because of fatigue
☐ Cannot because exercise makes symptoms worse

9. For the *past day* (past 24 hrs.), please rate the amount of perceived energy you have had using a scale from 0 to 100 where 0 = no energy and 100 = abundant energy:

_____

10. For the *past day* (past 24 hrs.), please rate the amount of energy you have expended (used) using a scale from 0 to 100 where 0 = no energy and 100 = all of your available energy:

_____

11. For the *past day* (past 24 hrs.), please rate the amount of fatigue you have had using a scale from 0 to 100 where 0 = no fatigue and 100 = severe fatigue:

_____

12. For the *past week,* please rate the amount of perceived energy you have had using a scale from 0 to 100 where 0 = none of your available energy and 100 = abundant energy:

_____

13. For the **past week,** please rate the amount of energy you have expended (used) using a scale from 0 to 100 where 0 = none of your available energy and 100 = all of your available energy:

   _____

14. For the **past week,** please rate the amount of fatigue you have had using a scale from 0 to 100 where 0 = no fatigue and 100 = severe fatigue:

   _____

15. How would you describe the course of your illness/health problems (check one)?

   ☐ Constantly getting worse
   ☐ Constantly improving
   ☐ Persisting (no change)
   ☐ Relapsing and remitting (having "good" periods with no symptoms and "bad" periods)
   ☐ Fluctuating (symptoms periodically wax and wane, but never disappear completely)

16. Do you have any known diagnosed medical conditions?

   _____

   _____

   _____

17. a.   Are you currently taking any medications (check one)?

   ☐ No     ☐ Yes

   b.   *If you replied "Yes" to 17a,* what medications are you taking?

   _____

   _____

   _____

18. How often do you drink alcohol (check one):

   ☐ Never      ☐ Rarely       ☐ Weekly        ☐ Daily

19. When you drink, how much do you typically drink?

_____

20. a.  Are you currently using recreational drugs (check one)?

    ☐ No    ☐ Yes

    b.  *If you replied "Yes" to 20a,* which drugs, how often, and how much do you use?

    _____

    _____

    _____

21. a.  Have you ever used recreational drugs in the past (check one)?

    ☐ No    ☐ Yes

    b.  *If you replied "Yes" to 21a,* which drugs, how often, and how much did you use?

    _____

    _____

    _____

22. a.  Have you ever been diagnosed or treated for an eating disorder (check one)?

    ☐ No    ☐ Yes

    b.  *If you replied "Yes" to 22a,* when did that problem begin?

    _____

    Do you still have an eating disorder (check one)?

    ☐ Yes    ☐ No

    When did the problem stop?

    _____

For the symptoms listed on the following pages, please indicate in the first column by placing a check ( ✓ ) by those symptoms that have persisted or reoccurred during 6 or more consecutive months of the fatigue illness.

In the next column, please place a check ( ✓ ) by those symptoms that began before you started having a persistent or recurring problem with fatigue.

In the third column, please indicate how often you have experienced any of the following symptoms *in the past 6 months* using these response categories: Never, seldom (about once a month or less), often or usually (occurs monthly), or always.

*In the last column please rate the severity of each symptom you have experienced **over the past 6 months** using a scale of 0 to 100 where 0 = no problem and 100 = the most severe problem possible.*

| Symptoms | Symptom Has Been Present for 6 Months or Longer | Symptom Began Before Fatigue Illness | Frequency (Never, Seldom, Often or Usually, or Always) | Symptom Severity Rating 0 to 100 |
|---|---|---|---|---|
| Fatigue | | | | |
| Sore Throat | | | | |
| Tender/Sore Lymph Nodes | | | | |
| Muscle Pain (That is, sensations of pain or aching in your muscles. This *does not* include weakness or pain in other areas such as joints.) | | | | |
| Pain in Multiple Joints Without Swelling or Redness | | | | |
| Impaired Memory or Concentration | | | | |
| Unrefreshing Sleep (That is, waking up feeling tired.) | | | | |

| Symptoms | Symptom Has Been Present for 6 Months or Longer | Symptom Began Before Fatigue Illness | Frequency (Never, Seldom, Often or Usually, or Always) | Symptom Severity Rating 0 to 100 |
|---|---|---|---|---|
| Postexertional Malaise, Feeling Worse After Doing Activities That Require Either Physical or Mental Exertion | | | | |
| Headaches* | | | | |

*IF EXPERIENCING HEADACHES:

Are these headaches you are experiencing more frequent, more severe, or in a different location than the headaches you experienced in the past before you began having problems with fatigue and your health (check all that apply)?

❒ More frequent     ❒ More severe     ❒ Different location

# CFS Screening Questionnaire

Date: _____ Phone Number: _____

## PART ONE
## THE CFS SCREENING QUESTIONNAIRE

START OF INTERVIEW

1. Would you be willing to answer a few questions now (check one)?

   ❏ Yes (Go to 2a.)   ❏ No

   *If no:*
   Can I call you back at a better time or schedule an appointment to talk to you (check one)?

   ❏ Yes (If yes, when? _____.)
   ❏ No

   *If no:*
   Caller should inquire why target is reluctant to participate. If so, caller should discuss special importance of their participation and should assure confidentiality and explain relevance and importance of studying fatigue.

   Reason for refusal:_____

First, I want to review some demographic information.

2.  a.   Do you live in the same home?

    ☐ Yes   ☐ No

    b.   Total number of household members (including yourself) who are 18 years
         of age or older:_____

3.  Your full name (in case we are cut off):

    First and Last Name _____

4.  Your Age Now? _____

5.  To which of the following U.S. census groups do you belong?

    ☐ African-American
    ☐ White
    ☐ Native American
    ☐ Asian or Pacific Islander
    ☐ Multiracial
    ☐ Other (specify):_____

6.  Are you of Latino or Hispanic origin?

    ☐ Yes   ☐ No

7.  Are you male or female?

    ☐ Female   ☐ Male

8.  Are you currently married, or are you separated, widowed, or divorced, or have
    you ever been married?

    ☐ Married
    ☐ Separated
    ☐ Widowed
    ☐ Divorced
    ☐ Never married

9.  Do you have any children?

    ☐ Yes (If yes, go to 10.)        ☐ No (If no, go to 11.)

10. How many children do you have? _____

11. What grade or degree have you completed in school?

❏ Less than high school
❏ Some high school
❏ High school degree or GED
❏ Partial college (at least 1 year) or specialized training
❏ Standard college degree
❏ Graduate professional degree including masters and doctorate

12. What is your current or most recent occupation?

Current:_____

Most recent:_____

---
NOTE: If currently unemployed, ask "Have you ever been employed?" If yes, record most recent job in "most recent" blank. If the person has never been employed, write "never employed" in the "most recent" blank.

---

[Do not read the items below. Just write in the occupation. If the person has never been employed, write "never employed" in the most recent blank.]

[Code Current or Most Recent Occupation Category After Interview.]

❏ Farm laborer/Menial service worker
❏ Unskilled worker
❏ Machine operator, semiskilled worker
❏ Skilled manual worker, craftsman, tenant farmer
❏ Clerical and sales worker
❏ Technician, semiprofessional, small-business owner
❏ Manager, minor professions
❏ Administrator, lesser professional, proprietor of medium-sized business
❏ Higher executive, proprietor of large business, major professional

13. Are you a:

|  | Yes | No |
|---|---|---|
| Student | ❏ | ❏ |
| Homemaker | ❏ | ❏ |
| Retired | ❏ | ❏ |
| Unemployed | ❏ | ❏ |
| Disabled | ❏ | ❏ |

14. What is your current work status?

   ❏ On disability (If on disability, go to 14a, all others go to 15.)
   ❏ Unemployed
   ❏ Working part-time
   ❏ Working full-time

   a. If on disability, for what condition do you receive disability compensation?
   Please specify: _____

[Items 15-25 are The Fatigue Scale, Chalder et al., 1993.*]

CALLER READS THE FOLLOWING: For the next few questions, we would like
to know whether you have had any problems with feeling tired, weak, or lacking in
energy in the last month. If you have been tired for a long time, we want you to
compare the way you feel now to how you felt when you were last well.

15. Do you have problems with tiredness?

   ❏ Less than usual
   ❏ No more than usual
   ❏ More than usual
   ❏ Much more than usual

16. Do you need to rest more?

   ❏ Less than usual
   ❏ No more than usual
   ❏ More than usual
   ❏ Much more than usual

17. Do you feel sleepy or drowsy?

   ❏ Less than usual
   ❏ No more than usual
   ❏ More than usual
   ❏ Much more than usual

---

*Reprinted from *Journal of Psychosomatic Research*, Vol. 17, No. 2, Chalder et al.,
"Development of a fatigue scale," pages 147-153, 1993, with permission from Elsevier
Science.

18. Do you have problems starting things?

   ❐ Less than usual
   ❐ No more than usual
   ❐ More than usual
   ❐ Much more than usual

19. Do you lack energy?

   ❐ Better than usual
   ❐ No more than usual
   ❐ More than usual
   ❐ Much more than usual

20. Do you have less strength in your muscles?

   ❐ Better than usual
   ❐ No more than usual
   ❐ More than usual
   ❐ Much more than usual

21. Do you feel weak?

   ❐ Less than usual
   ❐ Same as usual
   ❐ More than usual
   ❐ Much more than usual

22. Do you have difficulty concentrating?

   ❐ Less than usual
   ❐ Same as usual
   ❐ More than usual
   ❐ Much worse than usual

23. Do you find it more difficult to find the correct word?

   ❐ Less than usual
   ❐ No more than usual
   ❐ Worse than usual
   ❐ Much worse than usual

24. Do you make slips of the tongue when speaking?

    ❐ Less than usual
    ❐ No more than usual
    ❐ Worse than usual
    ❐ Much worse than usual

25. How is your memory?

    ❐ Better than usual
    ❐ No worse than usual
    ❐ Worse than usual
    ❐ Much worse than usual

26. Has fatigue, tiredness, or lack of energy caused

    ❐ No problems to your usual daily activities
    ❐ Minor problems to your usual daily activities
    ❐ Moderate problems to your usual daily activities
    ❐ Severe problems so that you are unable to perform your usual daily activities

27. Are you currently suffering from severe fatigue, extreme tiredness, or exhaustion that has been present for a period of 1 month or longer?

    ❐ Yes  ❐ No (If no, skip to 29.)

28. Are you currently suffering from severe fatigue, extreme tiredness, or exhaustion that has been present for a period of 6 months or longer?

    ❐ Yes  ❐ No

29. Do any other people in your household have severe fatigue, extreme tiredness, or exhaustion that has been present for a period of 6 months or longer?

    ❐ Yes  If yes, what are their names or initials? _____
    ❐ No (If No, skip to 30.)

---

The next few questions are designed to screen for (but not to diagnose) the overlapping chronic disorders of fibromyalgia and multiple chemical sensitivity (Donnay, 1998).*

---

*Reprinted with permission.

30. Compared to other people, would you say you are NOW

❐ More aware of odors than most
❐ About as aware of odors as most
❐ Less aware of odors than most
❐ More variable than most
❐ Don't know

31. Has that always been the case?

❐ No (If no, please answer 32a and 32b.)
❐ Yes (If yes, skip to question 33.)
❐ Don't know (If don't know, skip to question 33.)

32. a.  How did this change begin?

Gradually in 19____ / 20____
Suddenly in 19____ / 20____

b.  Do you associate this change with any event in your life?

❐ No
❐ Yes Check all that apply: ❐ Illness          ❐ Injury
                              ❐ Toxic Exposure ❐ Major Stress
                              ❐ Other, specify: _____

33. Over the last 6 months, how often have you deliberately tried to get away from or avoid being around particular odors because they made you feel ill?

❐ Don't Know
❐ Daily: at least once a day
❐ Weekly: not daily but at least once a week
❐ Monthly: not weekly, but at least once a month
❐ Rarely or never: less than once a month

34. Over the last month, how often have you felt feverish or had a fever?

❐ Don't know
❐ Daily: at least once a day
❐ Weekly: not daily but at least once a week
❐ Monthly: not weekly, but at least once in last month
❐ Not at all within the last 30 days

NOTE: In questions 35 and 36 below, "sick" refers to minor as well as more seri-ous health problems that can be physical or emotional.

35. How sick would you be if you had to fill your own gas tank?

❑ Not at all
❑ A little
❑ Moderately
❑ A lot
❑ Don't know

36. How sick would you be if you had to spend 4 hours in an enclosed shopping mall?

❑ Not at all
❑ A little
❑ Moderately
❑ A lot
❑ Don't know

37. Over the last 3 months, have you experienced chronic pain:

|  | Yes | No |
|---|---|---|
| a. Anywhere on the left side of your body | ❑ | ❑ |
| b. Anywhere on the right side of your body | ❑ | ❑ |
| c. Anywhere above your waist (anywhere in upper body or arms) | ❑ | ❑ |
| d. Anywhere below your waist (anywhere in lower body or legs) | ❑ | ❑ |
| e. Anywhere along your spine (from neck to lower back) | ❑ | ❑ |

Scoring of MCS and FMS screening questions can be found on page 128.

For those respondents who answered "No" to Question 27 (do not have 1+ months of fatigue) end here.

For those respondents who answered "Yes" to 28 (have fatigue 6+ months) go to 38.

## PART TWO—FOR RESPONDENTS WHO ANSWER YES TO 6 OR MORE MONTHS OF FATIGUE
### (see Question 28)

Now I would like to ask you some more specific questions about your fatigue.

38. How long have you had fatigue?

\_\_\_\_\_/_____ (yrs./mos.)

When did it begin? _____ (Specify the date, if possible.)

Over the last 6 months, to what degree have you experienced any of the following symptoms (Questions 39 to 52)?

39. Sore throat?

    ❒ Never
    ❒ Seldom
    ❒ Often or usually
    ❒ Always

40. Painful glands in your neck or under your arms?

    ❒ Never
    ❒ Seldom
    ❒ Often or usually
    ❒ Always

41. Muscle aches or pain?

    ❒ Never
    ❒ Seldom
    ❒ Often or usually
    ❒ Always

42. Do you feel generally worse than usual or fatigued for 24 hours or more after you have exercised?

    ❒ Never
    ❒ Seldom
    ❒ Often or usually
    ❒ Always

43. If you push yourself beyond your usual physical activity limits, do you feel worse than usual?

    ❒ Never
    ❒ Seldom
    ❒ Often or usually
    ❒ Always

44. Are you having headaches?

    ❒ Never (If never, skip to 46.)
    ❒ Seldom
    ❒ Often or usually
    ❒ Always

45. Are the headaches new or different from what you have experienced before the fatigue started?

   ❒ Never
   ❒ Seldom
   ❒ Often or usually
   ❒ Always

46. Do you have pain in your joints?

   ❒ Never
   ❒ Seldom
   ❒ Often or usually
   ❒ Always.

   Please specify which joints?_____

47. After a night's sleep, do you feel rested?

   ❒ Never
   ❒ Seldom
   ❒ Often or usually
   ❒ Always

48. After a night's sleep, does your fatigue go away temporarily?

   ❒ Never
   ❒ Seldom
   ❒ Often or usually
   ❒ Always

49. Are there times when you have had difficulty concentrating since the fatigue began?

   ❒ Never (If never, skip to 51.)
   ❒ Seldom
   ❒ Often or usually
   ❒ Always

50. Does your difficulty concentrating interfere with your work, study, or social activities?

   ❒ Never
   ❒ Seldom
   ❒ Often or usually
   ❒ Always

51. Are there times when you have trouble remembering things since the fatigue began?

   ☐ Never (If never, skip to 53.)
   ☐ Seldom
   ☐ Often or usually
   ☐ Always

52. Does your difficulty to remember things interfere with your work, study, or social activities?

   ☐ Never
   ☐ Seldom
   ☐ Often or usually
   ☐ Always

53. Are there other symptoms you have experienced during the past 6 months that were not mentioned in the previous questions (please specify)?

   _____

   _____

   _____

   _____

   _____

54. How frequently do you feel fatigued, tired, or lack energy?

   ☐ Not at all
   ☐ Less than once a week
   ☐ One to four times a week
   ☐ More than four times a week

55. Do you feel well, or greatly better, for days at a time?

   ☐ Yes   ☐ No (If no, skip to 57.)

56. Do you feel well, or greatly better, for weeks or more at a time?

   ☐ Yes   ☐ No

57. When your fatigue problem began, did it begin in

❒ Less than 24 hours
❒ 1 to 2 days
❒ 3 to 6 days
❒ 1 week to 1 month
❒ Longer than one month (Please specify the number months or years _____
_____.)
❒ Had fatigue since childhood or adolescence
❒ Don't know

58. Would you describe your fatigue problem as

❒ Getting worse over time
❒ Staying at about the same level
❒ Getting better over time

59. Do you experience high levels of fatigue or weakness following normal daily activity?

❒ Yes    ❒ No

60. Is your fatigue made worse by physical exertion (effort or activity)?

❒ Yes    ❒ No

61. Is your fatigue made worse by mental exertion (effort or activity)?

❒ Yes    ❒ No

62. Is your fatigue made worse by emotional distress?

❒ Yes    ❒ No

63. How long does it take the fatigue to begin after physical or mental exertion?

❒ Immediately
❒ About 1 hour
❒ From 1 to 3 hours
❒ More than 3 hours (Please specify number of hours _____.)

64. How long does the fatigue last after physical or mental exertion?

❏ One hour or less
❏ From 1 to 3 hours
❏ More than 3 hours (Please specify number of hours_____.)

65. Has your fatigue been present for more than 50% of the time?

❏ Yes   ❏ No

66. Which of the following statements best describes your fatigue during the *last month?*

❏ I am not able to work or do anything, and I am bedridden.
❏ I can walk around the house, but I cannot do light housework.
❏ I can do light housework, but I cannot work part-time.
❏ I can only work part-time at work or on some family responsibilities.
❏ I can work full-time, but I have no energy left for anything else.
❏ I can work full-time and finish some family responsibilities, but I have no energy left for anything else.
❏ I can do all work or family responsibilities without any problems with my energy.

67. a.   Have you ever consulted a medical doctor about your fatigue problem?

❏ Yes (Go to b.)
❏ No (Go to 69.)

b.   Has your doctor told you what she or he thinks is causing the fatigue?

Specify:_____

68. Do you currently have a medical doctor overseeing your fatigue problems?

❏ Yes   ❏ No

69. Has a doctor ever diagnosed you with any of the following illnesses? (If yes, ask respondent to provide date of diagnosis.)

Yes No

a. ☐ ☐ Date: _____ Current heart or heart valve infection
b. ☐ ☐ Date: _____ Congestive heart failure
c. ☐ ☐ Date: _____ Stroke causing paralysis or problems with speech or thinking
d. ☐ ☐ Date: _____ Asthma using steroid medications (current)
e. ☐ ☐ Date: _____ Emphysema
f. ☐ ☐ Date: _____ TB (current)
g. ☐ ☐ Date: _____ Hepatitis (current)
h. ☐ ☐ Date: _____ Cirrhosis (current or lifetime)
i. ☐ ☐ Date: _____ Kidney disease (current)
j. ☐ ☐ Date: _____ Multiple sclerosis (current or lifetime)
k. ☐ ☐ Date: _____ Myasthenia gravis (current or lifetime)
l. ☐ ☐ Date: _____ Epilepsy or seizures (uncontrolled)
m. ☐ ☐ Date: _____ Lupus (current or lifetime)
n. ☐ ☐ Date: _____ Diabetes (untreated only)
o. ☐ ☐ Date: _____ Cancer other than skin (current)
p. ☐ ☐ Date: _____ Polymyositis/Dermatomyositis
q. ☐ ☐ Date: _____ Rheumatoid arthritis
r. ☐ ☐ Date: _____ HIV/AIDS
s. ☐ ☐ Date: _____ Schizophrenia of any kind
t. ☐ ☐ Date: _____ Bipolar affective disorders
u. ☐ ☐ Date: _____ Depression with psychotic or melancholic feature
v. ☐ ☐ Date: _____ Delusional or psychotic disorder of any kind
w. ☐ ☐ Date: _____ Dementia of any kind
x. ☐ ☐ Date: _____ Anorexia nervosa
y. ☐ ☐ Date: _____ Bulimia nervosa
z. ☐ ☐ Date: _____ Untreated hypothyroidism
aa. ☐ ☐ Date: _____ Sleep apnea
bb. ☐ ☐ Date: _____ Narcolepsy
cc. ☐ ☐ Date: _____ Side effects of medications (e.g., drowsiness)
dd. ☐* ☐ Date: _____ Alcohol, drug, or other substance abuse within 2 years before onset of the chronic fatigue and at any time afterward

---

*If yes to substance abuse, when did it begin? Specify date:_____.
If yes, are you still abusing alcohol? ☐ Yes ☐ No
If no, when did you stop? Specify date: _____.

---

70. Do you have any other previously diagnosed medical illnesses or conditions which may still be active and causing chronic fatigue (e.g., pregnancy or menopause)?

    ❏ Yes (If yes, please specify _____.)
    ❏ No

---

NOTE: If the respondent answered yes to any items in 69 or named any condition in 70, list each illness or condition below and ask the questions that follow. If there are more than two illnesses, continue on another sheet. If respondent did not report any illnesses or conditions in 69 and 70, skip to 72a.

---

71. a. Illness #1:_____    b. Illness #2:_____

| | |
|---|---|
| Do you feel Illness #1 is causing your fatigue? | Do you feel Illness #2 is causing your fatigue? |
| ❏ All of the fatigue<br>❏ Some of the fatigue<br>❏ Not causing the fatigue | ❏ All of the fatigue<br>❏ Some of the fatigue<br>❏ Not causing the fatigue |
| When did Illness #1 begin compared to the start of your fatigue? | When did Illness #2 begin compared to the start of your fatigue? |
| Did it begin: | Did it begin: |
| ❏ Before the fatigue<br>❏ The same time as the fatigue<br>❏ After the fatigue | ❏ Before the fatigue<br>❏ The same time as the fatigue<br>❏ After the fatigue |
| Is Illness #1 being successfully treated? | Is Illness #2 being successfully treated? |
| ❏ Yes<br>❏ No (If no, skip to rating below.) | ❏ Yes<br>❏ No (If no, skip to rating below.) |
| Rate how effective this treatment is in decreasing your fatigue on a scale from 0 to 100 (0 = Not at all effective and 100 = Completely effective)?_____ | Rate how effective this treatment is in decreasing your fatigue on a scale from 0 to 100 (0 = Not at all effective and 100 = Completely effective)?_____ |

72.  a.  Do you think any medication(s) is(are) causing your fatigue? (If more than two, continue on another sheet)

❏ Yes (If yes, please specify below.)
❏ No (If no, skip to 73a.)

b.  Medication #1:_____     c.  Medication #2:_____

What is the approximate
dosage?

_____

How often do you take this
dosage?

_____

Do you feel it is causing your
fatigue?

❏ All of the fatigue
❏ Some of the fatigue
❏ Not causing the fatigue

What is the approximate
dosage?

_____

How often do you take this
dosage?

_____

Do you feel it is causing your
fatigue?

❏ All of the fatigue
❏ Some of the fatigue
❏ Not causing the fatigue

73.  a.  Do you think anything else accounts for your fatigue problems? For example, being overworked, depressed, or stressed in your personal life or environment?

❏ Yes  Please specify:_____
❏ No

b.  To what degree do you feel these factors account for your fatigue:

❏ All of the fatigue
❏ Some of the fatigue
❏ Not causing the fatigue

74.  a.  Can your fatigue be explained by ongoing strenuous physical activity?

❏ Yes
❏ No

b.  To what degree do you feel this ongoing strenuous physical activity accounts for your fatigue:

❏ All of the fatigue
❏ Some of the fatigue
❏ Not causing my fatigue

75. Do you have a history of allergies?

   ❐ Yes  ❐ No

76. With extended rest, does your chronic fatigue and all its symptoms go away?

   ❐ Yes, for a long period of time
   ❐ Yes, for a short period of time
   ❐ No, not at all

77. I would like to know what you think is causing your fatigue problems. Do you feel the cause is:

   ❐ Definitely physical
   ❐ Mainly physical
   ❐ Equally physical and psychological
   ❐ Mainly psychological
   ❐ Definitely psychological

78. a.  What is your height? _____

    b.  What is your weight? _____

# Other CFS Symptoms

For the symptoms below, please indicate in the first column by placing a check ( ✓ ) by those symptoms that have persisted or reoccurred during 6 or more consecutive months of the fatigue illness.

In the next column please check ( ✓ ) those symptoms that began before you started having a persistent or recurring problem with fatigue.

In the third column please indicate how often you have experienced any of the following symptoms *in the past 6 months* using these response categories: Never, seldom (about once a month or less), often or usually (occurs monthly), or always.

In the last column please rate the severity of each symptom you have experienced *over the past 6 months* using a scale of 0 to 100 where 0 = no problem and 100 = the most severe problem possible.

| | Symptom Has Been Present for 6 Months or Longer | Symptom Began Before Fatigue Illness | Frequency (Never, Seldom, Often or Usually, or Always) | Symptom Severity Rating 0 to 100 |
|---|---|---|---|---|

*Physical Complaints*

| | | | | |
|---|---|---|---|---|
| Racing heart | | | | |
| Chest pain | | | | |
| Shortness of breath | | | | |
| Upset stomach | | | | |
| Nausea | | | | |
| Sensitivity to alcohol | | | | |

| | Symptom Has Been Present for 6 Months or Longer | Symptom Began Before Fatigue Illness | Frequency (Never, Seldom, Often or Usually, or Always) | Symptom Severity Rating 0 to 100 |
|---|---|---|---|---|
| Abdomen pain | | | | |
| Weight change | | | | |
| Poor appetite | | | | |
| Dizziness | | | | |
| Ringing in the ears | | | | |
| Sweating hands | | | | |
| Night sweats | | | | |
| Tense muscles | | | | |
| Chilled or shivery | | | | |
| Hot or cold spells | | | | |
| Feeling like you have a temperature | | | | |
| Fevers | | | | |

| | Symptom Has Been Present for 6 Months or Longer | Symptom Began Before Fatigue Illness | Frequency (Never, Seldom, Often or Usually, or Always) | Symptom Severity Rating 0 to 100 |
|---|---|---|---|---|
| Temperature lower than normal | | | | |
| Tingling feeling | | | | |
| Paralysis | | | | |
| Blurred vision | | | | |
| Abnormal sensitivity to light | | | | |
| Blind spots | | | | |
| Eye pain | | | | |
| Rash | | | | |
| Allergies | | | | |
| Chemical sensitivity | | | | |
| Muscle weakness | | | | |
| Feel unsteady on feet | | | | |
| Need to nap during each day | | | | |

| | Symptom Has Been Present for 6 Months or Longer | Symptom Began Before Fatigue Illness | Frequency (Never, Seldom, Often or Usually, or Always) | Symptom Severity Rating 0 to 100 |
|---|---|---|---|---|
| Difficulty falling asleep | | | | |
| Difficulty staying asleep | | | | |
| Waking up early in the morning (e.g., 3 a.m.) | | | | |
| Difficulty staying asleep | | | | |
| Other: | | | | |

**Other Cognitive Difficulties**

| | | | | |
|---|---|---|---|---|
| Slowness of thought | | | | |
| Absent-Mindedness | | | | |
| Confusion/ Disorientation | | | | |
| Difficulty reasoning things out | | | | |

|  | Symptom Has Been Present for 6 Months or Longer | Symptom Began Before Fatigue Illness | Frequency (Never, Seldom, Often or Usually, or Always) | Symptom Severity Rating 0 to 100 |
|---|---|---|---|---|
| Forgetting what you are trying to say |  |  |  |  |
| Difficulty finding the right word |  |  |  |  |
| Difficulty following things |  |  |  |  |
| Difficulty compre-hending information |  |  |  |  |
| Need to have to focus on one thing at a time |  |  |  |  |
| Frequently lose train of thought |  |  |  |  |
| Trouble expressing thoughts |  |  |  |  |
| Difficulty retaining information |  |  |  |  |
| Difficulty recalling information |  |  |  |  |
| Frequently get words or numbers in the wrong order |  |  |  |  |

| | Symptom Has Been Present for 6 Months or Longer | Symptom Began Before Fatigue Illness | Frequency (Never, Seldom, Often or Usually, or Always) | Symptom Severity Rating 0 to 100 |
|---|---|---|---|---|
| Slow to react | | | | |
| Poor hand-to-eye coordination | | | | |
| New trouble with math | | | | |
| Concern with driving | | | | |
| Other: | | | | |

### Mood Difficulties

| | | | | |
|---|---|---|---|---|
| Anxiety/Tension | | | | |
| Easily irritated | | | | |
| Depression | | | | |
| Mood swings | | | | |
| Other: | | | | |

Scoring of MCS Screening Items (Questions 31, 34, 35, & 36) (Donnay, 1998).

Positive screen for MCS requires M > 0 where M = the sum of variously weighted responses to Questions 31, 34, 35, and 36 as defined below. The M statistic was developed by Johns Hopkins researchers Dr. Penelope Keyl and Dr. Ann Davidoff. Confirmation of the MCS diagnosis still requires a complete history and physical exam.

Calculating "M": An MCS diagnosis is unlikely if M is negative and likely if M is positive where:
$$M = (3.97*A) + (4.94*B) + (2.37*C) + (1.29*D) - 6.21$$

and:

A = Q31 score: Yes = 0, No = 1, Don't know = 0
B = Q34 score: Daily or Weekly = 1, Monthly or Not at all = 0, Don't know = 0
C = Q35 score: No = 0, A little = 1, Moderately = 2, A lot = 3, Don't know = 0.5
D = Q36 score: No = 0, A little = 1, Moderately = 2, A lot = 3, Don't know = 0.5

Scoring of FMS Screening Item (Question 37) (Donnay, 1998).

Positive screen for FMS requires Question 37a to Question 37e = Yes. Confirmation of the FMS diagnosis still requires finding at least 11 of 18 specific tender points on physical exam.

# Fatigue-Related Cognitions Scale*

Name: _____ Date: _____

Below is a series of statements regarding your fatigue. By fatigue we mean a sense of tiredness, lack of energy, or total body give-out.

In the past 2 weeks, my average level of fatigue was (circle one):

|   1   |   2   |   3   |   4   |   5   |   6   |   7   |   8   |   9   |   1 0  |
|-------|-------|-------|-------|-------|-------|-------|-------|-------|-------|
| Very Mild Fatigue | | | | Moderate Fatigue | | | | Severe Fatigue | |

---

Please indicate the extent to which you agree or disagree with each of the statements below using the following 5-point scale. Please answer these questions as they apply to the past 2 weeks.

> 1 = Disagree Strongly
> 2 = Disagree Moderately
> 3 = Neither Agree Nor Disagree
> 4 = Agree Moderately
> 5 = Agree Strongly

_____        1.    I think about my fatigue often.

_____        2.    I worry if I will be cured of my fatigue.

_____        3.    My fatigue makes me angry.

_____        4.    I need support from family or friends to cope with my fatigue.

_____        5.    It is awful to feel as fatigued as I do.

_____        6.    I sometimes think I deserve the fatigue I feel.

_____        7.    I can't get rid of my fatigue.

_____        8.    I have no control over my fatigue.

_____        9.    I sometimes think I'm dying because my fatigue symptoms are so severe.

_____        10.   Fatigue is very frustrating for me.

_____        11.   I sometimes have suicidal thoughts due to my fatigue.

_____        12.   My fatigue-related limitations make me feel guilty.

_____        13.   I feel sorry for myself as a fatigue victim.

_____        14.   My fatigue helps me get the attention I feel I deserve.

# Fennell Phase Inventory*

Please indicate the extent to which you agree or disagree with each of the statements below using the following 5-point scale.

> 1 = Definitely Do Not Agree
> 2 = Do Not Agree
> 3 = Somewhat Agree
> 4 = Agree
> 5 = Very Strongly Agree

_____ 1. I feel like I am falling apart. (a)

_____ 2. I am just beginning to recognize when and how my symptoms occur. (b)

_____ 3. I am beginning to accept the fact that I will never be completely like I was before the illness and that I will need to become a new person. (b)

_____ 4. I now have learned that living with the illness involves getting sicker, at times, and improving, at times. (c)

---

*Note. From "An Investigation of the Different Phases of the CFS Illness," by L. A. Jason, P. A. Fennell, S. Klein, G. Fricano, J. A. Halpert, and R. R. Taylor, 1999, *The Journal of Chronic Fatigue Syndrome, 5,* pp. 53-54. Copyright © 1999 by the Haworth Press, Inc. Reprinted with permission.

_____    5.    The primary way for me to improve is if my physician finds me the right treatment. (a)

_____    6.    I am beginning to seek the support and information from others who have or who know about the illness. (b)

_____    7.    I am in the early process of creating meaning about my illness experience. (b)

_____    8.    I have gained a sense of myself that is blended—a combination of my life before and after I first got sick. (c)

_____    9.    I need to know with certainty when and if I am going to get better. (a)

_____    10.   I am just starting to feel like I have some control of my life. (b)

_____    11.   I am beginning to learn how to live with the unknown or chronic nature of my illness. (b)

_____    12.   I have better and more satisfying relationships with people I care about since I first became sick. (d)

_____    13.   It is my fault I got sick. (d)

_____    14.   I am just starting to realize that there may be things I can do to help myself feel better. (b)

_____    15.   I am starting to see my illness experience as having some value. (b)

_____    16.   I am proud of myself for living with this illness. (c)

_____    17.   I think about my illness all of the time. (a)

_____    18.   I am just beginning to stabilize (i.e., feeling a bit less confused and a bit more ordered). (b)

_____    19.   For the first time, I am beginning to have compassion and love for myself and for what I have endured. (b)

_____    20.   I am a better and wiser person since I first got sick. (c)

a = Crisis Factor
b = Stabilization Factor
c = Integration Factor
d = Item Did Not Significantly Load

# Scoring Key for Fennell Phase Inventory

The Crisis mean score was calculated by adding Items 1, 5, 9, and 17 of the Fennell Phase Inventory and dividing by 4. The Stabilization mean score was calculated by adding Items 2, 3, 6, 7, 10, 11, 14, 15, 18, and 19 of the Fennell Phase Inventory and dividing by 10. The Integration mean score was calculated by adding Items 4, 8, 16, and 20 of the Fennell Phase Inventory and dividing by 4.

These scoring criteria are in Jason, Fricano, et al. (2000). Using Crisis, Stabilization, and Integration mean scores (see above), each participant was then assigned to one of the four groups according to the following algorithmic criteria derived from the cluster analysis from the data in the Jason, Fennell, et al. (1999) study. Criteria for the Crisis group were a Crisis score of 3.00 or above and Stabilization and Integration scores of 3.30 or below. Criteria for the Integration group were a Crisis score of 2.50 or below, a Stabilization score of 2.80 or below, and an Integration score of 4.25 or above. Cases not in either of these groups that had either a Crisis score of 3.10 or above, a Stabilization score of 3.40 or above, or an Integration score of 3.75 or above were classified into a Resolution group. Cases that did not meet any of the above criteria comprised the Stabilization group.

These four cluster scores parallel the four phases of Fennell's (1993) model. In Phase 1, the individual with CFS moves into a crisis mode shortly after illness onset, wherein he or she experiences the traumatic aspects of a new illness. In Phase 2, the person with CFS continues to experience chaos and dissembling, followed by the eventual stabilization of symptoms. In Phase 3, the person with CFS moves into the resolution mode, as he or she works to accept the chronicity and ambiguity of this chronic illness and create meaning out of the illness experience. Finally, in Phase 4, the person with CFS achieves integration, wherein he or she is able to integrate pre- and post-illness self-concepts and respond to the illness in a more planful way.

| SCORING KEY | | | |
|---|---|---|---|
| **Phase Categories** | **Crisis Score** | **Stabilization Score** | **Integration Score** |
| Crisis Phase | $\geq 3.0$ | $\leq 3.3$ | $\leq 3.3$ |
| Stabilization Phase | If case doesn't meet any of criteria for other phases | | |
| Resolution Phase | $\geq 3.10$ | $\geq 3.4$ | $\geq 3.75$ |
| Integration Phase | $\leq 2.5$ | $\leq 2.8$ | $\geq 4.25$ |

# The Chronic Fatigue Syndrome Attitudes Test Questions*

Please indicate the extent to which you agree or disagree with each of the following statements using the following 7-point scale:

> 1 = Strongly Disagree
> 2 = Disagree
> 3 = Slightly Disagree
> 4 = Neither Agree Nor Disagree
> 5 = Slightly Agree
> 6 = Agree
> 7 = Strongly Agree

_____  1.  Children with CFS should be allowed to attend regular classes.

_____  2.  Employers should be permitted to fire those with CFS.

_____  3.  People with CFS are just depressed.

---

*Note. Adapted from "The Development of the Chronic Fatigue Syndrome Attitudes Test," by J. L. Shlaes, L. A. Jason, and J. R. Ferrari, 1999, *Evaluation and the Health Professionals, 22*(4), pp. 442-465. Copyright © 1999 by Sage Publications, Inc. Reprinted by permission of Sage Publications, Inc.

_____   4.   More federal funds should be allocated for research on CFS.

_____   5.   People with CFS are lazy.

_____   6.   I would continue to visit and support a friend who has CFS.

_____   7.   People with CFS should not be discriminated against in any way.

_____   8.   CFS is not a real medical illness.

_____   9.   I would shake hands with someone with CFS.

_____  10.   The majority of people with CFS were competitive, driven to achieve, and compulsive before they got sick.

_____  11.   I would not sit on the same toilet that a person with CFS had just used.

_____  12.   CFS is not as big a problem as the media suggests.

_____  13.   People with CFS would get better if they really wanted to be healthy.

_____  14.   CFS is primarily a psychological disorder.

_____  15.   The majority of people with CFS have a high socioeconomic status.

_____  16.   CFS is one of the leading medical problems in the country.

_____  17.   If people with CFS rest, then they will get better.

_____  18.   People with CFS are to blame for getting sick.

_____  19.   CFS is a form of punishment from God.

For scoring purposes, use only Items 2, 3, 4, 5, 8, 10, 11, 12, 13, 14, 17, 18, and 19 (reverse score Item 4). You can sum these items for an overall composite score and also add up the items below to use the following three factor scores:

| | |
|---|---|
| Responsibility for CFS: | Items 3, 5, 11, 18, 19 |
| Relevance of CFS: | Items 2, 4, 8, 12 |
| Traits of People With CFS: | Items 10, 13, 14, 17 |

# Behavioral Rating Scales

## Symptom/Affect/Activity Record Form

The record form that follows includes ratings on a 0 to 100 numerical rating scale of the following subjective states: perceived energy, expended energy, fatigue, positive feelings, and negative feelings. Zero (0) represents a complete absence of the subjective state and 100, the presence of the subjective state as strong as it could be. As explained to patients, **perceived energy** refers to the level of energy one experiences at any particular moment. **Expended energy** refers to the amount of energy used up at any particular moment, while **fatigue** refers to a sense of generalized tiredness. **Positive feelings** indicate the sum total of all positive feelings (e.g., happiness, elation) and **negative feelings** refer to the sum total of all negative feelings (e.g., sadness, anxiety).

In the **Daily Activities** column, patients are asked to highlight specific mental and physical activities during each specific 2-hour block (e.g., phone conversation, housekeeping, childcare, etc.). In addition, to get an objective measure of physical activity, the clinician can obtain (or ask the client to obtain) an electronic step-counter (pedometer) which is worn on the beltline at all times except when bathing or sleeping. (We use a Radio Shack step-counter which costs about $12.) The device records the number of **steps taken** during ordinary locomotion. Clients are instructed to record the number of steps displayed on the device each time they rated their subjective states during the 2-hour block.

During the first or second session, patients are asked to complete the record form for 7 to 14 consecutive days with entries made 6 times a day at approximately 2-hour intervals beginning in the morning after awakening. Each entry is made on the record form and can be completed at any time within each consecutive 2-hour period.

The completed record form will help the clinician and the patient to evaluate the relationships between activities, symptoms, and emotional states. Patterns that may be found include overwork/collapse, negative affect/higher symptom severity, positive affect/lower symptom severity, and so forth. Once identified, a collaborative plan between clinician and patient can be developed to modify symptom-exacerbating patterns (see Chapters 6 and 7).

# Daily Energy and Fatigue Record*

0 = Least     100 = Most          Day/Date _____

| Perceived Energy (energy you have) | Expended Energy (energy used up) | Fatigue | Positive Feelings | Negative Feelings | Daily Activities | Steps Taken |
|---|---|---|---|---|---|---|
|  |  |  |  |  |  |  |
|  |  |  |  |  |  |  |
|  |  |  |  |  |  |  |
|  |  |  |  |  |  |  |
|  |  |  |  |  |  |  |
|  |  |  |  |  |  |  |
|  |  |  |  |  |  |  |

*Note. From "Chronic Fatigue Syndrome and Fibromyalgia: Clinical Assessment and Treatment," by F. Friedberg and L. A. Jason, in press, *Journal of Clinical Psychology*. Copyright by the American Psychological Association. Reprinted with permission.

# Resources for Individuals With CFS, FMS, and MCS

## Chronic Fatigue Syndrome

National support groups providing information and support for individuals with CFS, including referrals for local area support groups, health care providers specializing in CFS, and up-to-date information regarding medical research:

*CFIDS Association of America, Inc.*
P.O. Box 220398
Charlotte, NC 28222-0398
Phone: 800-442-3437
Website: www.cfids.org

*The National CFIDS Foundation, Inc.*
103 Aletha Road
Needham, MA 02492
Phone: 781-449-3535
Fax: 781-449-8606
Website: www.ncf-net.org

*National Chronic Fatigue Syndrome and Fibromyalgia Association*
P.O. Box 18426
Kansas City, MO 64133
Phone: 816-313-2000

### *CFS Websites:*

*Author Leonard Jason's CFS Home Page*
http://condor.depaul.edu/~ljason/cfs

*American Association for Chronic Fatigue Syndrome*
http://www.aacfs.org/

*The CFIDS Association of America*
http://www.efids.org

*Chicago CFS Association*
http://www.enteract.com/~choward/

*R.E.D.D. or Rnase-L Enzyme Dysfunction Disease,* is based on research by Robert Suhadolnik. According to this theory, a low molecular weight (LMW) 2' - 5' A binding polypeptide (37kDa) is produced instead of the normal 80kDa protein. It is possible that LMW RnaseL functions as a strong binder for the RNA that the body produces to fight viruses–and in fact it binds the RNA out of the process altogether. The result is that the essential last stage in the body's antiviral defense pathway is missing. To find out more, look at the R.E.D.D. home page: http://www.cfids-me.org/redd/

*The CFS Radio Show*
http://www.cfsaudio.4biz.net/cfsradio.htm

*CFIDS/Fibromyalgia Self-Help Program*
Book: CFIDS/Fibromyalgia Toolkit
http://www.cfidsselfhelp.org

*CFIDS & Fibromyalgia Health Resource*
http://www.healthresource.com

*Chronic Immunological and Neurological Diseases Association (CINDA)*
http://www.cinda.org

*Educational Rights of Young Persons With CFS*
http://www.wicknet.com/hosting/cfids

*Frank Albrecht's Website: "For Parents of Sick and Worn-Out Kids"*
http://home.bluecrab.org/~health/sickids.html

*Website for CFIDS & Fibromyalgia Health Resource*
A good source of health information and high quality vitamins and supplements.
http://www.immunesupport.com

An informational website and mailing list designed to promote effective distribution and exchange of information between medical/clinical, political, and patient communities.
http://www.Co-Cure.org

## Fibromyalgia

*F.A.C.E.S. INC. Fibromyalgia Association Created for Education and Self-Help*
A network of self-help groups in the Chicago metropolitan area.
Email: fibrocop@hotmail.com
Phone: 773-731-1228
Website: http://hometown.aol.com/fibrocop1/myhomepage/profile.html

*Fibromyalgia Network*
A national support organization for individuals with FMS that publishes an informative newsletter.
P.O. Box 31750
Tucson, AZ 85751-1750
Phone: 520-290-5508
Website: http://www.fmnetnews.com

### *Fibromyalgia Websites:*

*The Fibromyalgia Association of Greater Washington*
http://www.Fmagw.org

*Fibromyalgia Network News*
http://www.FMNetNews.com

*The National Fibromyalgia Awareness Campaign*
http://www.FMAware.com

*The Fibromyalgia Alliance of America*
http://www.FMAA.org

*The Oregon Fibromyalgia Foundation*
http://www.Myalgia.com

*Information Clearing Houses*
http://www.Fibromyaliga.com
http://www.Hellingwell.com
http://www.plaidrabbit.com

## Multiple Chemical Sensitivities

*Multiple Chemical Sensitivity Referral and Resources, Inc.*
Provides outreach, resources for health care professionals, patient support, and public advocacy.
508 Westgate Road
Baltimore, MD 21229-2343
Phone: 410-362-6400
Fax: 410-362-6401
Email: donnaya@rtk.net
Website: www.mcsrr.org

*EI/MCS Support*
Publishes Canary News, an informative newsletter dedicated to MCS issues.
1404 Judson Avenue
Evanston, IL 60201
Phone: 847-866-9630

The following companies offer catalogues and sell a variety of environmentally safe products for individuals with multiple chemical sensitivities and other allergic conditions, including nontoxic cleaning supplies, clothing, household paint, and air filters:

*National Ecological and Environmental Delivery System (N.E.E.D.S.)*
527 Charles Avenue, 12-A
Syracuse, NY 13209
Phone: 800-634-1380
Fax: 800-295-6333

*Allergy Control Products, Inc.*
96 Danbury Road
Ridgefield, CT 06877
Phone: 800-422-3878
Fax: 203-431-8963

# Other Resources for Individuals
# With CFS, FMS, and MCS

*Information About the Americans With Disabilities Act Can Be Found At:*
U.S. Department of Justice
Civil Rights Division
Public Access Section
P.O. Box 65860
Washington, DC 20277-1806
Phone: 800-232-9675

*National Information Center for Children and Youth With Disabilities*
P.O. Box 1492
Washington, DC 20013
Phone: 202-884-8200

*Food Stamps*
Phone: 800-252-8635

*Handicapped Parking Placard*
Phone: 800-252-8980

*Social Security Administration*
Phone: 800-772-1213

*Social Security Disability Hotline*
Phone: 800-637-8856

*Frequently Asked Questions on Social Security Disability*
Website: http://www.nosscr.org

# References

American Psychiatric Association. (1994). *Diagnostic and Statistical Manual of Mental Disorders* (4th ed.). Washington, DC: Author.

Amir, M., Neumann, L., Bor, O., Shir, Y., Rubinow, A., & Buskila, D. (2000). Coping styles, anger, social support, and suicide risk of women with fibromyalgia syndrome. *Journal of Musculoskeletal Pain, 8,* 7-20.

Anderson, J. S., & Ferrans, C. E. (1997). The quality of life of persons with chronic fatigue syndrome. *Journal of Nervous and Mental Disease, 185,* 359-367.

Ang, D., & Wilkes, W. S. (1999). Diagnosis, etiology, and therapy of fibromyalgia. *Comprehensive Therapy, 25,* 221-227.

Bartha, L., Baumzweiger, W., Buscher, D. S., Callender, T., Dahl, K. A., Davidoff, A., Donnay, A., Edelson, S. B., Elson, B. D., Elliot, E., Flayhan, D. P., Heuser, G., Keyl, P. M., Kilburn, K. H., Gibson, P., Jason, L. A., Krop, J., Mazlen, R. D., McGill, R. G., McTamney, J., Meggs, W. J., Morton, W., Nass, M., Oliver, L. C., Panjwani, D. D., Plumlee, L. A., Rapp, D., Shayevitz, M. B., Sherman, J., Singer, R. M., Solomon, A., Vodjani, A., Woods, J. M., & Ziem, G. (1999). Multiple chemical sensitivity: A 1999 consensus. *Archives of Environmental Health, 54,* 147-149.

Bartley, S. H., & Chute, E. (1969). *Fatigue and Impairment in Man.* New York: Johnson Reprints.

Beck, A. J. (1967). *Depression: Clinical, Experimental and Theoretical Aspects.* New York: Harper & Row.

Bell, I. R., Baldwin, C. M., & Schwartz, G. E. (1998). Illness from low levels of environmental chemicals: Relevance to chronic fatigue syndrome and fibromyalgia. *American Journal of Medicine, 105,* 74S-82S.

Bell, I. R., Rossi, J., Gilbert, M. E., Kobal, G., Morrow, L. A., Newlin, D. B., Sorg, B. A., & Wood, R. W. (1997). Testing the neural sensitization and kindling hypothesis for illness from low level environmental chemicals. *Environmental Health Perspectives, 105*(Suppl. 2), 539-547.

Blenkiron, P., Edwards, R., & Lynch, S. (1999). Associations between perfectionism, mood, and fatigue in chronic fatigue syndrome: A pilot study. *Journal of Nervous and Mental Disorders, 187,* 566-570.

Blumer, D., & Heilbronn, M. (1981). The pain-prone disorder: A clinical and psychological profile. *Psychosomatics, 22,* 395-397, 401-402.

Buchwald, D., & Garrity, D. (1994). Comparison of patients with chronic fatigue syndrome, fibromyalgia, and multiple chemical sensitivity. *Archives of Internal Medicine, 154,* 2049-2053.

Buchwald, D., Pearlman, T., Umali, J., Schmaling, K., & Katon, W. (1996). Functional status in patients with chronic fatigue syndrome, other fatiguing illnesses, and healthy individuals. *American Journal of Medicine, 101*(4), 364-370.

Chalder, T., Berelowitz, G., Pawlikowska, T., Watts, L., Wessely, S., Wright, D., & Wallace, E. P. (1993). Development of a fatigue scale. *Journal of Psychosomatic Medicine, 37*(2), 147-153.

Consensus Document on Fibromyalgia: The Copenhagen Declaration. (1992, August 17-20). Issued by the Second World Congress on Myofascial Pain and Fibromyalgia meeting. Published *Lancet,* Vol. 340, Sept. 12, 1992, and incorporated into the World Health Organization's 10th revision of the *International Statistical Classification of Diseases and Related Health Problems, ICD 10,* Jan. 1, 1993. Available from Bente Danneskiold-Samsoe, Department of Rheumatology, Fredriksberg Hospital, Ndr Fasanvej 57, DK-2000 Frederiksberg, Denmark. Also in the *Journal of Musculoskeletal Pain,* Vol. 1, No. 3/4, 1993.

Cullen, M. R. (1987). Multiple chemical sensitivities: Summary and directions for future investigations. *Occupational Medicine, 2*(4), 801-804.

Davis, T. H., Jason, L. A., & Banghart, M. A. (1998). The effect of housing on individuals with multiple chemical sensitivities. *Journal of Primary Prevention, 19,* 31-42.

Deale, A., Chalder, T., Marks, I., & Wessely, S. (1997). Cognitive behaviour therapy for chronic fatigue syndrome: A randomized controlled trial. *American Journal of Psychiatry, 154,* 408-414.

Dechene, L., Friedberg, F., MacKenzie, M., & Fontanetta, R. (1994). *A New Fatigue Typology for Chronic Fatigue Syndrome.* Unpublished manuscript.

DeLuca, J., Johnson, S. K., Ellis, S. P., & Natelson, B. H. (1997). Sudden versus gradual onset of chronic fatigue syndrome differentiates individuals on cognitive and psychiatric measures. *Journal of Psychiatric Research, 31,* 83-90.

Demitrack, M. A., Dale, J. K., Straus, S. E., Laue, L., Listwak, S. J., Kreusi, M. J. P., Chrousos, G. P., & Gold, P. W. (1991). Evidence for impaired activation of the hypothalamic-pituitary-adrenal axis in patients with chronic fatigue syndrome. *Journal of Clinical Endocrinology and Metabolism, 72*(6), 1-11.

Donnay, A. (1998, April 29). *Questionnaire for Screening CFS, FMS, and MCS in Adults.* Testimony presented to the U.S. CFS Coordinating Committee, Washington, DC.

Donnay, A., & Ziem, G. (1998, October). *Prevalence and Overlap of Chronic Fatigue Syndrome and Fibromyalgia Syndrome Among 100 New Patients With Multiple Chemical Sensitivity Syndrome.* Paper presented at the American Association of Chronic Fatigue Syndrome Research Conference, Cambridge, MA.

Ellis, A. (1997). Using rational emotive behavior therapy techniques to cope with disability. *Professional Psychology: Research and Practice, 28,* 17-22.

Fennell, P. A. (1993). A systematic, four-stage progressive model for mapping the CFIDS experience. *The CFIDS Chronicle, Summer,* 40-46.

Ferrans, C. E. (1990). Quality of life: Conceptual issues. *Seminars in Oncology Nursing, 6*(4), 248-254.

Ferrans, C. E., & Powers, M. J. (1985). Quality of life index: Development and psychometric properties. *Advances in Nursing Science, 8*(1), 15-24.

Ferrans, C. E., & Powers, M. J. (1992). Psychometric assessment of the Quality of Life Index. *Research in Nursing and Health, 15*, 29-38.

Field, T. M. (1998). Massage therapy effects. *American Psychologist, 53*, 1270-1281.

First, M. B., Spitzer, R. L., Gibbon, M., & Williams, J. B. W. (1995). *Structured Clinical Interview for DSM-IV Axis I Disorders — Patient Edition.* New York: Biometrics Research Department.

Forsyth, L. M., Preuss, H. G., MacDowell, A. L., Chiazze, L., Birkmayer, G. D., & Bellanti, J. A. (1999). Therapeutic effects of oral NADH on the symptoms of patients with chronic fatigue syndrome. *Annals of Allergy, Asthma, and Immunology, 82*, 185-191.

Friedberg, F. (1995). *Coping With Chronic Fatigue Syndrome: Nine Things You Can Do.* Oakland, CA: New Harbinger.

Friedberg, F. (1996). Chronic fatigue syndrome: A new clinical application. *Professional Psychology: Research and Practice, 27*, 487-494.

Friedberg, F. (1999). A subgroup analysis of cognitive-behavioral treatment studies. *Journal of Chronic Fatigue Syndrome, 5*, 149-159.

Friedberg, F. (2000). *A Subgroup Analysis in Chronic Fatigue Syndrome: A Time Series Analysis.* Manuscript submitted for publication.

Friedberg, F., Dechene, L., McKenzie, M., & Fontanetta, R. (2000). Symptom patterns in long-duration chronic fatigue syndrome. *Journal of Psychosomatic Research, 48*, 59-68.

Friedberg, F., & Jason, L. A. (1998). *Understanding Chronic Fatigue Syndrome: An Empirical Guide to Assessment and Treatment.* Washington, DC: American Psychological Association.

Friedberg, F., & Jason, L. A. (in press). Chronic fatigue syndrome and fibromyalgia: Clinical assessment and treatment. *Journal of Clinical Psychology.*

Friedberg, F., & Krupp, L. B. (1994). A comparison of cognitive behavioral treatment for chronic fatigue syndrome and primary depression. *Clinical Infectious Diseases, 18*(Suppl. 1), S105-S110.

Friedberg, F., McKenzie, M., Dechene, L., & Fontanetta, R. (1994, October). *Symptom Patterns in Long-Term Chronic Fatigue Syndrome.* Paper presented at the American Association of Chronic Fatigue Syndrome Research Conference, Ft. Lauderdale, FL.

Fukuda, K., Straus, S. E., Hickie, I., Sharpe, M. C., Dobbins, J. G., & Komaroff, A. (1994). The chronic fatigue syndrome: A comprehensive approach to its definition and study. *Annals of Internal Medicine, 121*, 953-959.

Goldberg, D. P. (1972). *The Detection of Psychiatric Illness by Questionnaire.* Oxford, England: Oxford University Press.

Granges, G., & Littlejohn, G. O. (1993). A comparative study of clinical signs in fibromyalgia/fibrositis syndrome, healthy and exercising subjects. *Journal of Rheumatology, 20*(2), 344-351.

Guglielmi, R. S., Cox, D. J., & Spyker, D. A. (1994). Behavioral treatment of phobic avoidance in multiple chemical sensitivity. *Journal of Behavior Therapy and Experimental Psychiatry, 25*(3), 197-209.

Haley, R. W, & Kurt, T. L. (1997). Self-reported exposure to neurotoxic chemical combinations in the Gulf War: A cross-sectional epidemiologic study. *Journal of the American Medical Association, 277*(3), 231-237.

Haley, R. W., Kurt, T. L., & Hom, J. (1997). Is there a Gulf War syndrome? *Journal of the American Medical Association, 277*(3), 215-222.

Hay, A.W. M., Jaffer, S., & Davies, D. (2000). Chronic exposure to carbon monoxide: A neglected problem. *European Journal of Oncology, 5,* 25-33.

Hickie, I., Bennett, B., Lloyd, A., Heath, A., & Martin, N. (1999). Complex genetic and environmental relationships between psychological distress, fatigue and immune functioning: A twin study. *Psychological Medicine, 29,* 267-277.

Hickie, I., & Davenport, T. (1999). The case of Julio: A behavioral approach based on reconstructing the sleep-wake cycle. *Cognitive and Behavioral Practice, 6,* 442-450.

Holmes, G. P., Kaplan, J. E., Gantz, N. M., Komaroff, A. L., Schonberger, L. B., Strauss, S. S., Jones, J. F., Dubois, R. E., Cunningham-Rudles, C., Pahwa, S., Tosato, G., Zegans, L. S., Purtilo, D. T., Brown, W., Schooley, R. T., & Brus, I. (1988). Chronic fatigue syndrome: A working case definition. *Annals of Internal Medicine, 108,* 387-389.

Jason, L. A., Fennell, P. A., Klein, S., Fricano, G., Halpert, J. A., & Taylor, R. R. (1999). An investigation of the different phases of the CFS illness. *Journal of Chronic Fatigue Syndrome, 5,* 35-54.

Jason, L. A., Ferrari, J. R., Taylor, R. R., Slavich, S. P., & Stenzel, C. L. (1996). A national assessment of the service, support, and housing preferences by persons with chronic fatigue syndrome: Toward a comprehensive rehabilitation program. *Evaluation and the Health Professions, 19,* 194-207.

Jason, L. A., Fricano, G., Taylor, R. R., Halpert, J., Fennell, P. A., Klein, S., & Levine, S. (2000). Chronic fatigue syndrome: An examination of the phases. *Journal of Clinical Psychology, 56,* 1497-1508.

Jason, L. A., King, C. P., Richman, J. A., Taylor, R. R., Torres, S. R., & Song, S. (1999). U.S. case definition of chronic fatigue syndrome: Diagnostic and theoretical issues. *Journal of Chronic Fatigue Syndrome, 5*(3), 3-33.

Jason, L. A., Melrose, H., Lerman, A., Burroughs, V., Lewis, K., King, C. P., & Frankenberry, E. L. (1999). Managing chronic fatigue syndrome: A case study. *American Association of Occupational Health Nurses Journal, 47,* 17-21.

Jason, L. A., Richman, J. A., Rademaker, A. W., Jordan, K. M., Plioplys, A. V., Taylor, R. R., McCreedy, W., Huang, C., & Plioplys, S. (1999). A community-based study of chronic fatigue syndrome. *Archives of Internal Medicine, 159,* 2129-2137.

Jason, L. A., Ropacki, M. T., Santoro, N. B., Richman, J. A., Heatherly, W., Taylor, R., Ferrari, J. R., Plioplys, A. V., Plioplys, S., Rademaker, A., & Golding, J. (1997). A screening scale for chronic fatigue syndrome: Reliability and validity. *Journal of Chronic Fatigue Syndrome, 3,* 39-59.

Jason, L. A., Taylor, R. R. & Kennedy, B. A. (2000). Chronic fatigue syndrome, fibromyalgia, and multiple chemical sensitivities in a community-based sample of persons with chronic fatigue syndrome-like symptoms. *Psychosomatic Medicine, 62,* 655-663.

Jason, L. A., Taylor, R. R., Plioplys, S., Stepanek, Z., & Shlaes, J. (in press). Evaluating attributions for an illness based upon the name: Chronic fatigue syndrome, myalgic encephalopathy and florence nightingale disease. *American Journal of Community Psychology.*

Jason, L. A., Taylor, R. R., Stepanek, Z., & Plioplys, S. (in press). Attitudes regarding chronic fatigue syndrome: The importance of a name. *Journal of Health Psychology.*

Jason, L. A., Tryon, W., Frankenberry, E., & King, C. (1997). Chronic fatigue syndrome: Relationships of self-ratings and actigraphy. *Psychological Reports, 81,* 1223-1226.

Jason, L. A., Wagner, L., Taylor, R., Ropacki, M. T., Shlaes, J., Ferrari, J., Slavich, S. P., & Stenzel, C. (1995). Chronic fatigue syndrome: A new challenge for health care professionals. *Journal of Community Psychology, 23,* 143-164.

Johnson, S. K., DeLuca, J., & Natelson, B. (1999). Chronic fatigue syndrome: Reviewing the research findings. *Annals of Behavioral Medicine, 21,* 258-271.

Joyce, J., Hotopf, M., & Wessely, S. (1997). The prognosis of chronic fatigue and chronic fatigue syndrome: A systematic review. *Quarterly Journal of Medicine, 90,* 223-233.

Kansky, G. (2000). Is Ampligen a death sentence? *The National Forum, 3,* 14-15.

King, C. P., Jason, L. A., Frankenberry, E. L., Tryon, W. W., & Jordan, K. M. (1997). Management of chronic fatigue syndrome through behavioral monitoring of energy levels and fatigue. *CFIDS Chronicle, 10,* 10-14.

Komaroff, A. L., Fagioli, L. R., Geiger, A. M., Doolittle, T. H., Lee, J., Kornish, J., Gleit, M. A., & Guerriero, R. T. (1996). An examination of the working case definition of chronic fatigue syndrome. *American Journal of Medicine, 100,* 56-64.

Kreutzer, R., Neutra, R. R., & Lashuay, N. (1999). Prevalence of people reporting sensitivities to chemicals in a population-based survey. *American Journal of Epidemiology, 150*(1), 1-12.

Krupp, L. B., LaRocca, N. G., Muir-Nash, J., & Steinberg, A. D. (1989). The Fatigue Severity Scale. *Archives of Neurology, 46,* 1121-1123.

Lapp, C. W. (1992). Chronic fatigue syndrome is a real disease. *North Carolina Family Physician, 43,* 6-11.

Lawson, L. (1993). *Staying Well in a Toxic World.* Chicago: The Noble Press.

LeRoy, J., Haney Davis, T., & Jason, L. A. (1996). Treatment efficacy: A survey of 305 MCS patients. *The CFIDS Chronicle, Winter,* 52-53.

Lloyd, A. R., Hickie, I., Boughton, C. R., Spencer, O., & Wakefield, D. (1990). Prevalence of chronic fatigue syndrome in an Australian population. *Medical Journal of Australia, 153,* 522-528.

McHorney, C. A., Ware, J. E., Lu, R. L., & Sherbourne, D. (1994). The MOS 36-Item Short-Form Health Survey (SF-36): III. Tests of data quality, scaling assumptions, and reliability across diverse patient groups. *Medical Care, 32*(1), 40-66.

McHorney, C. A., Ware, J. E., & Raczek, A. E. (1993). The MOS 36-Item Short Form Health Survey (SF-36): II. Psychometric and clinical tests of validity in measuring physical and mental health constructs. *Medical Care, 31*(3), 247-263.

Medical Outcomes Trust. (1994). *How to Score the SF-36 Health Survey.* Boston: Author.

Miller, C. S. (1992). Possible models for multiple chemical sensitivity: Conceptual issues and role of the limbic system. *Toxicology and Industrial Health, 8,* 181-202.

Pepper, C. M., Krupp, L. B., Friedberg, F., Doscher, C., & Coyla, P. K. (1993). A comparison of neuropsychiatric characteristics in chronic fatigue syndrome, multiple sclerosis, and major depression. *The Journal of Neuropsychiatry and Clinical Neurosciences, 5,* 200-205.

Pesek, J. R., Jason, L. A., & Taylor, R. R. (2000). An empirical investigation of the envelope theory. *Journal of Human Behavior in the Social Environment, 3,* 59-77.

Plioplys, S., & Plioplys, A. V. (1995). Chronic fatigue syndrome. *Southern Medical Journal, 88,* 993-1000.

Ray, C., Jefferies, S., & Weir, W. R. C. (1995). Coping with chronic fatigue syndrome: Illness responses and their relationship with fatigue, functional impairment and emotional status. *Psychological Medicine, 25,* 937-945.

Ray, C., Weir, W. R. C., Stewart, D., Miller, P., & Hyde, G. (1993). Ways of coping with chronic fatigue syndrome: Development of an illness management questionnaire. *Social Science Magazine, 37,* 385-391.

Reid, S., Chalder, T., Cleare, A., Hotopf, M., & Wessely, S. (2000). Extracts from "clinical evidence": Chronic fatigue syndrome. *British Medical Journal, 320,* 292-296.

Robins, L., Helzer, J., Cottler, L., & Goldring, E. (1989). *National Institute of Mental Health Diagnostic Interview Schedule, Version Three Revised. DIS-III-R.* St. Louis, MO: Department of Psychiatry, Washington University School of Medicine.

Ross, P. M., Whysner, J., Covello, V. T., Kuschner, M., Rifkind, A. B., Sedler, M. J., Trichopoulos, D., & Williams, G. M. (1999). Olfaction and symptoms in the multiple chemical sensitivities syndrome. *Preventive Medicine, 28*(5), 467-480.

Rossy, L. A., Buckelew, S. P., Dorr, N., Hagglund, K. J., Thayer, J. F., McIntosh, M. J., Hewett, J. E., & Johnson, J. C. (1999). A meta-analysis of fibromyalgia treatment interventions. *Annals of Behavioral Medicine, 21,* 180-191.

Schwartz, R. B., Komaroff, A. L., Garada, B. M., Gleit, M., Doolittle, T. H., Bates, D. W., Vasile, R. G., & Holman, B. L. (1994). SPECT imaging of the brain: Comparisons of findings in patients with chronic fatigue syndrome, AIDS dementia complex, and major unipolar depression. *American Journal of Radiology, 162,* 943-951.

Sharpe, M. C., Archard, L. C., Banatvala, J. E., Borysiewicz, L. K., Clare, A. W., David, A., Edwards, R. H. T., Hawton, K. E. H., Lambert, H. P., Lane, R. J. M., McDonald, E. M., Mowbray, J. F., Pearson, D. J., Peto, T. E. A., Preedy, V. R., Smith, A. P., Smith, D. G., Taylor, D. J., Tyrrell, D. A. J., Wessely, S., & White, P. D. (1991). A report — chronic fatigue syndrome: Guidelines for research. *Journal of the Royal Society of Medicine, 84,* 118-121.

Sharpe, M. C., Hawton, K. E. H., Simkin, S., Surawy, C., Hackmann, A., Klimes, I., Peto, T., Warrell, D., & Seagroatt, V. (1996). Cognitive behaviour therapy for the chronic fatigue syndrome: A randomized controlled trial. *British Medical Journal, 312,* 22-26.

Shlaes, J. L., Jason, L. A., & Ferrari, J. R. (1999). The development of the Chronic Fatigue Syndrome Attitudes Test. *Evaluation and the Health Professions, 22*(4), 442-465.

Starlanyl, D., & Copeland, M. E. (1996). *Fibromyalgia and Chronic Myofascial Pain Syndrome.* Oakland, CA: New Harbinger.

Suhadolnik, R. J., Reichenbach, N. L., Hitzges, P., Adelson, M. E., Peterson, D. L., Cheney, P., Salvato, P., Thompson, C., Loveless, M., Muller, W. E. G., Schroder, H. C., Strayer, D., & Carter, W. (1994). Changes in the 2-5A synthetase/Rnase L antiviral pathway in a controlled clinical trial with Poly(I)-Poly(C12U) in chronic fatigue syndrome. *In Vivo, 8,* 599-604.

Suhadolnik, R. J., Reichenbach, N. L., Hitzges, P., Sobol, R. W., Peterson, D. L., Henry, B., Ablashi, D. V., Muller, W. E., Schroder, H. C., Carter, W. A., & Strayer, D. R. (1994). Upregulation of the 2-5A synthetase/Rnase L antiviral pathway associated with chronic fatigue syndrome. *Clinical Infectious Diseases, 18*(1), S96-S104.

Surawy, C., Hackmann, A., Hawton, K., & Sharpe, M. (1995). Chronic fatigue syndrome: A cognitive approach. *Behavior Research and Therapy, 33,* 535-544.

Taylor, R. R., & Jason, L. A. (1998). Comparing the DIS with the SCID: Chronic fatigue syndrome and psychiatric comorbidity. *Psychology and Health: The International Review of Health Psychology, 13,* 1087-1104.

Taylor, R. R., Jason, L. A., & Torres, A. (2000). Fatigue rating scales: An empirical comparison. *Psychological Medicine, 30,* 849-856.

Vercoulen, J. H. M. M., Swanink, C. M. A., Zitman, F. G., Vreden, G. S., & Hoofs, M. P. E. (1996). Randomized, double-blind, placebo-controlled study of fluoxetine in chronic fatigue syndrome. *The Lancet, 347,* 858-862.

Verrillo, E. F., & Gellman, L. M. (1997). *Chronic Fatigue Syndrome: A Treatment Guide.* New York: St. Martin's Griffin.

Ware, J. E., & Sherbourne, C. D. (1992). The Medical Outcomes Study 36-Item Short-Form Health Survey (SF-36): Conceptual framework and item selection. *Medical Care, June,* 473-483.

Waylonis, G. W., & Perkins, R. H. (1994). Post-traumatic fibromyalgia: A long-term follow-up. *American Journal of Physical Medicine and Rehabilitation, 73,* 403-412.

Weiss, B. (1997). Experimental strategies for research on multiple chemical sensitivity. *Environmental Health Perspectives, 105*(2), 487-494.

Wessely, S. (1998). The epidemiology of chronic fatigue syndrome. *Epidemiologia e Psichiatria Sociale, 7*(1) 19-24.

White, K. P., Harth, M., Speechley, M., & Ostbye, T. (1999). Testing an instrument to screen for fibromyalgia syndrome in general population studies: The London Fibromyalgia Epidemiology Study Screening Questionnaire. *Journal of Rheumatology, 26*(4), 880-884.

Wolfe, F., Ross, K., Anderson, J., Russell, I. J., & Hebert, L. (1995). The prevalence and characteristics of fibromyalgia in the general population. *Arthritis and Rheumatism, 38*(1), 19-28.

Wolfe, F., Smythe. H. A., Yunus, M. B., Bennett, R. M., Bombardier, C., Goldenberg, D. L., Tugwell, P., Campbell, S. M., Abeles, M., Clark, P., Fam, A. G., Farber, S. J., Fiewchtner, J. J., Franklin, C. M., Gatter, R. A., Hamaty, D., Lessard, J., Lichtbroun, A. S., Masi, A. T., McCain, G. A., Reynolds, W. J., Romano, T. J., Russell, I. J., & Sheon, R. P. (1990). The American College of Rheumatology 1990 criteria for the classification of fibromyalgia. *Arthritis and Rheumatology, 33,* 160-172.

# Subject Index

# Author Index

## A

Adelson, 14, 53
American Psychiatric Association (APA), 31, 32
Amir, 22
Anderson, 4, 45
Ang, 16

## B

Baldwin, 2
Banghart, 6
Bartha, 6
Bartley, 42
Beck, 47
Bell, 2, 18
Blenkiron, 14
Blumer, 21
Buchwald, 27, 44

## C

Chalder, 42, 43, 69, 108
Chute, 42
Copeland, 5, 52, 55
Cox, 22
Cullen, 19

# If You Found This Book Useful . . .

You might want to know more about our other titles.

If you would like to receive our latest catalog, please return this form:

Name: _____
(Please Print)

Address: _____

Address: _____

City/State/Zip: _____
This is ☐ home ☐ office

Telephone: (_____) _____

E-mail: _____

I am a:

☐ Psychologist                    ☐ Marriage and Family Therapist
☐ Psychiatrist/Physician          ☐ Patient
☐ Nurse                           ☐ Not in Health Care Field
☐ Clinical Social Worker          ☐ Other: _____
☐ Mental Health Counselor

◆          ◆          ◆

**Professional Resource Press**
**P.O. Box 15560**
**Sarasota, FL  34277-1560**

**Telephone: 800-443-3364**
**FAX:  941-343-9201**
**E-mail: mail@prpress.com**
**Website: http://www.prpress.com**

CI/4/01(Behavmed)

# Add A Colleague To Our Mailing List . . .

If you would like us to send our latest catalog to one of your colleagues, please return this form:

Name: _____
(Please Print)

Address: _____

Address: _____

City/State/Zip: _____
This is ☐ home ☐ office

Telephone: (_____)_____

E-mail: _____

This person is a:

☐ Psychologist                    ☐ Marriage and Family Therapist
☐ Psychiatrist/Physician          ☐ Patient
☐ Nurse                           ☐ Not in Health Care Field
☐ Clinical Social Worker          ☐ Other: _____
☐ Mental Health Counselor

Name of person completing this form: _____

◆          ◆          ◆

**Professional Resource Press**
**P.O. Box 15560**
**Sarasota, FL  34277-1560**

**Telephone: 800-443-3364**
**FAX:  941-343-9201**
**E-mail: mail@prpress.com**
**Website: http://www.prpress.com**

CI/4/01(Behavmed)

# If You Found This Book Useful . . .

You might want to know more about our other titles.

If you would like to receive our latest catalog, please return this form:

Name: _____
(Please Print)

Address: _____

Address: _____

City/State/Zip: _____
This is ☐ home ☐ office

Telephone: (_____) _____

E-mail: _____

I am a:

☐ Psychologist                    ☐ Marriage and Family Therapist
☐ Psychiatrist/Physician          ☐ Patient
☐ Nurse                           ☐ Not in Health Care Field
☐ Clinical Social Worker          ☐ Other: _____
☐ Mental Health Counselor

◆        ◆        ◆

**Professional Resource Press**
**P.O. Box 15560**
**Sarasota, FL  34277-1560**

**Telephone: 800-443-3364**
**FAX:  941-343-9201**
**E-mail: mail@prpress.com**
**Website: http://www.prpress.com**

# Add A Colleague To Our Mailing List . . .

If you would like us to send our latest catalog to one of your colleagues, please return this form:

Name: _____
(Please Print)

Address: _____

Address: _____

City/State/Zip: _____
This is  ❏ home   ❏ office

Telephone: (_____) _____

E-mail: _____

This person is a:

❏  Psychologist                     ❏  Marriage and Family Therapist
❏  Psychiatrist/Physician           ❏  Patient
❏  Nurse                            ❏  Not in Health Care Field
❏  Clinical Social Worker           ❏  Other: _____
❏  Mental Health Counselor

Name of person completing this form: _____

◆          ◆          ◆

**Professional Resource Press**
**P.O. Box 15560**
**Sarasota, FL  34277-1560**

**Telephone: 800-443-3364**
**FAX:  941-343-9201**
**E-mail: mail@prpress.com**
**Website: http://www.prpress.com**

CI/4/01(Behavmed)

616

101027

T2455